Midwifery Essentials
Postnatal

For Elsevier:

Commissioning Editor: Mairi McCubbin
Development Editor: Sheila Black
Project Manager: Christine Johnston
Designer: Charlotte Murray, Kirsteen Wright
Illustrations Manager: Merlyn Harvey

Midwifery Essentials

Volume 4 **Postnatal**

Helen Baston BA(Hons) MMedSci PhD PGDipEd ADM RN RM

Lead Midwife for Education; Supervisor of Midwives, Mother & Infant Research Unit, Department of Health Sciences, University of York, York, UK

Jennifer Hall MSc ADM PGDip(HE) RN RM

Senior Lecturer in Midwifery, Faculty of Health and Life Sciences, University of the West of England, Bristol, UK

Foreword by

Julie Wray MSc PGCHE ADM RN RM ONC

Iolanthe Research Fellowship 2008; Senior Lecturer and Service User/Carer Lead, School of Nursing, Faculty of Health and Social Care, University of Salford, Salford, UK

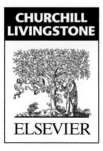

Edinburgh   London   New York   Oxford   Philadelphia   St Louis   Sydney   Toronto   2009

CHURCHILL
LIVINGSTONE
ELSEVIER

First published 2009

ISBN 978-0-443-10356-8

British Library Cataloguing in Publication Data
A catalogue record for this book is available from the British Library

Library of Congress Cataloging in Publication Data
A catalog record for this book is available from the Library of Congress

Notice
Knowledge and best practice in this field are constantly changing. As new research and experience broaden our knowledge, changes in practice, treatment and drug therapy may become necessary or appropriate. Readers are advised to check the most current information provided (i) on procedures featured or (ii) by the manufacturer of each product to be administered, to verify the recommended dose or formula, the method and duration of administration, and contraindications. It is the responsibility of the practitioner, relying on their own experience and knowledge of the patient, to make diagnoses, to determine dosages and the best treatment for each individual patient, and to take all appropriate safety precautions. To the fullest extent of the law, neither the Publisher nor the Editors assumes any liability for any injury and/or damage to persons or property arising out or related to any use of the material contained in this book.

Printed in China

Contents

When I reflect back on my own midwifery training in the 1980s I am struck by the lack of theory and minimal literature dedicated to postnatal care. This is something that has always bemused me, considering that midwives have had almost exclusivity within postnatal practice and that they lead within this aspect of childbirth. Interestingly, some years later, in 1997, the Audit Commission highlighted that many women in England and Wales found postnatal care to be the least satisfying aspect of their maternity care experiences. Profoundly, it took women who participated in the Audit Commissions survey to highlight difficulties with postnatal care provision. For the most part the hospital stay featured more negatively but nevertheless this finding rang alarm bells within maternity care and the midwifery profession.

In parallel, evidence emerged to support the notion that postnatal care is often viewed as a low priority amongst midwives (Bondas-Salonen 1998). Clearly a dissonance between the profession and women's experience has existed for many years. A contributing factor could arguably be a lack of supporting literature to underpin and guide practice. Most recently maternity care policy,

including NICE guidelines, has however, attempted to address the evidence void by producing specific guidance for practice, which is very welcome, and this policy context is referred to in the book.

I am delighted that Helen Baston and Jenny Hall have taken the initiative and put together a practical, easy-to-read, unique book on postnatal care. This book has huge potential for learning. Both student midwives and practising midwives will benefit, as will the women and families for whom they care.

From my own perspective, postnatal care has had much appeal and I have enjoyed working in this area. I have published papers questioning the use of the metaphor 'Cinderella' in connection with postnatal care, as have others, and have undertaken research in this area. It was in 2003 that I first wrote in *The Practising Midwife* about my concerns regarding postnatal care (Wray 2003) and Helen Baston published a useful paper on postnatal care under the auspice of Midwifery basics in 2004 (Baston 2004). Interestingly, in the April 2009 issue of the journal, the front cover headlined 'The Cinderella service: postnatal care', which infers as Jenny Hall has said that 'nothing has changed'. Thus the publication of this book is extremely pertinent and places postnatal care on the map. It emphasises best practice and offers a useful model, the Jigsaw Model, to inform, guide and underpin postnatal practice.

It is my pleasure and honour to recommend this contemporaneous book and hope that like me you will find it very useful, enlightening and thus a core text for midwifery – enjoy!

Salford, 2009

Julie Wray

References

Baston H: Midwifery basics: postnatal care, principles and practice, *The Practising Midwife* 7(11):40–45, 2004.

Bondas-Salonen T: New mothers' experiences of postnatal care – a phenomenological follow-up study, *Journal of Clinical Nursing* 7:165–174, 1998.

Wray J: Do we care or is it an afterthought? Postnatal care–the good and the bad, *The Practising Midwife* 6(4):4–5, 2003.

To contribute to the provision of sensitive, safe and effective maternity care for women and their families is a privilege. Childbirth is a life-changing event for women. Those around them and those who input into any aspect of pregnancy, labour, birth or the postnatal period can positively influence how this event is experienced and perceived. In order to achieve this, maternity carers continually need to reflect on the services they provide and strive to keep up-to-date with developments in clinical practice. They should endeavour to ensure that women are central to the decisions made and that real choices are offered and supported by skilled practitioners.

This book is the fourth volume in a series of texts based on the popular 'Midwifery Basics' series published in *The Practising Midwife* journal. Since their publication, there have been many requests from students, midwives and supervisors to combine the articles into a handy text to provide a resource for learning and refreshment of midwifery knowledge and skills. The books have remained true to the original style of the articles and have been updated and expanded to create a user-friendly source of information. They are also intended to stimulate debate and require the reader both to reflect on their current practice, local policies

and procedures and to challenge care that is not woman-centred. The use of scenarios enables the practitioner to understand the context of maternity care and explore their role in its safe and effective provision.

There are many dimensions to the provision of woman-centred care that practitioners need to consider and understand. To aid this process, a jigsaw model has been introduced, with the aim of encouraging the reader to explore maternity care from a wide range of perspectives. For example, how does a midwife obtain consent from a woman for a procedure, maintain a safe environment during the delivery of care and make the most of the opportunity to promote health? What are the professional and legal issues in relation to the procedure and is this practice based on the best available evidence? Which members of the multi-professional team contribute to this aspect of care and how is it influenced by the way care is organized? Each aspect of the jigsaw should be considered during the assessment, planning, implementation and evaluation of woman-centred maternity care.

Midwifery Essentials: Postnatal is about the provision of safe and effective postnatal care. It comprises ten chapters, each written to stand alone or be read in succession. The introductory chapter sets the scene, exploring the role of the midwife in the context of professional and national guidance. The jigsaw model for midwifery care is introduced and explained, providing a framework to explore each aspect of postnatal care, described in subsequent chapters. Chapter 2 explores the principles and practice of postnatal care. It describes the common features of the postnatal examination of the woman and the examination of the baby performed by the midwife. Chapter 3 focuses on the care of the baby in the immediate postnatal period and describes the features of the normal neonate. Chapter 4 goes on to detail the newborn clinical examination that is performed by the paediatrician (and increasingly the midwife/nurse who has undergone further education) within the first 72 hours of life. Chapter 5 focuses on hospital postnatal care and

Chapter 6 builds on this, examining the specific needs of women who have undergone caesarean section. In Chapter 7 the role of the community midwife in the provision of postnatal care at home is discussed, followed by Chapter 8, which focuses on postnatal emotional wellbeing. In Chapter 9, the issues around postnatal fertility control are described, including physiological as well as pharmacological methods. The book concludes with Chapter 10, which explores the issues involved in supporting a woman to feed her baby. This book thoroughly prepares the reader to provide safe, evidence-based, woman-centred postnatal care for mothers and their babies.

Helen Baston

York and Bristol, 2009   Jennifer Hall

Acknowledgements

In the process of writing there are always people behind the scenes who support or add to the development of the book. We would specifically like to thank Mary Seager, formerly Senior Commissioning Editor at Elsevier, for her initial vision, support and prompting to turn the journal articles from *The Practising Midwife* into a readable volume. In addition, neither of us could have completed this project without the love, support, patience and endless cups of tea and coffee provided by our partners and children. To you we owe our greatest gratitude.

Chapter 1

Introduction

This book is the fourth in the *Midwifery Essentials* series aimed at student midwives and those who support them in clinical practice. It focuses on postnatal care for low-risk women beginning with the principles and practice of postnatal midwifery care. It then considers care of the neonate immediately after the birth, followed by full physical examination of the newborn. Postnatal care of the mother is described in the hospital, after caesarean birth and then in the community setting. Consideration is then given to emotional wellbeing after birth and fertility control. The book concludes with an exploration of how the new mother can be supported to feed her baby. Scenarios are used throughout the book to facilitate learning and assist the reader to apply this knowledge to her own practice areas. The focus for contemporary maternity care is choice, access and continuity of care within a safe and effective service (Department of Health 2004, 2007). This book

explores ways in which this aspiration can become a reality for women and their families.

The aim of this introductory chapter is:

- To introduce the 'jigsaw model' for exploring effective midwifery practice.

The jigsaw model is used throughout the book with a view to helping midwives apply their knowledge in the provision of woman-centred postnatal care.

Midwifery care model

One of the purposes of this series of books is to consider the care of women and their babies from an holistic viewpoint. This means considering the care from a physical, emotional, psychological, spiritual, social and cultural context. To do this we have developed a jigsaw model of care that will encourage the reader to consider individual aspects of midwifery care, while recognizing that these aspects go to make up part of the whole person being cared for.

This model will be used to reflect on the clinical scenarios described in the chapters. It shows the dimensions of effective maternity care and each should be considered during the assessment, planning, implementation and evaluation of an aspect of care.

The pieces of the jigsaw clearly interlink with each other and each is needed for the provision of safe, holistic postnatal care. When one is missing the picture will be incomplete and care will not reach its potential. Each aspect of the model is described below in more detail. It is recommended that when an aspect of midwifery care is being evaluated that each piece of the jigsaw is addressed. Consider the questions pertaining to each piece of the jigsaw and work through those that are relevant to the clinical situation you face.

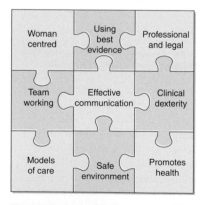

Fig. 1.1 Jigsaw model: dimensions of effective midwifery care.

Woman-centred care

The provision of woman-centred care was one of the central messages of the policy document *Changing childbirth* (Department of Health 1993) which turned the focus of maternity care from meeting the needs of the professionals to listening and responding to the aspirations of women. This is further enforced in the *National Service Framework* (Department of Health 2004) and *Maternity matters* (Department of Health 2007) and the National Institute for Health and Clinical Excellence (NICE) *Postnatal care guidelines* (NICE 2006). The provision of woman-centred care is also an expectation of midwifery practice (NMC 2004) and pre-registration education (NMC 2009). When considering particular aspects of care the questions that need to be addressed to ensure that the woman's care is woman-centred include:

- Was the woman involved in the development of her postnatal care plan and its subsequent implementation?
- Did the woman have a choice about where she accessed her postnatal care?
- Is this care designed to meet the woman's needs or that of the service?
- How can I ensure that she remains involved in further decisions about her care?
- What are the implications of undertaking or not undertaking this examination on this particular woman and baby?

- Are there any factors that I need to consider that might influence the results of this examination for this woman and their impact on her?
- How does this package of postnatal care fit in with the woman's hopes, expectations and meanings?
- Is now the most appropriate time to undertake this aspect of care?

Using best evidence

There is a growing body of research evidence that is available to inform the postnatal care we provide. We have a duty to apply this knowledge, as the NMC Code states: 'you must deliver care based on the best available evidence or best practice' (NMC 2008:4). Midwifery evidence includes many aspects (Wickham 2004) and the decisions a midwife makes about her practice will be influenced by a range of factors. However, in the statement above, care should be based as much as possible on the 'best' evidence, whatever that is. Questions that need to be addressed when exploring the evidence base of care include:

- What is already known about this aspect of care?
- What is the justification for the choices made about care?
- What is the research evidence available on this examination?
- Do local guidelines reflect best evidence?
- Was a midwife involved in development of local/national guidelines?

- Who represents users of maternity services on groups where guidelines are developed?
- What midwifery research project has your Trust been involved in, in relation to postnatal care?
- Where do you go first in order to identify sources of best evidence?

Professional and legal

Women need to feel confident that the midwives who care for them are working within a framework that supports safe practice. Midwives who practise in the United Kingdom must adhere to the rules and guidance of the Nursing and Midwifery Council (NMC). The Code (NMC 2008:01) states:

As a professional you are accountable for actions and omissions in your practice and must always justify your decisions. You must always act lawfully, whether those laws relate to your professional practice or personal life.

Midwives are therefore required to comply with English law and the rules and regulations of their employers.

Questions that need to be addressed to ensure that the woman's care fulfils statutory obligations include:

- Is this procedure expected to be an integral part of education prior to qualification?
- How do the midwives rules relate to this care?
- Which NMC proficiencies relate to this care?

- How does the NMC Code relate to this care?
- Is there any other NMC guidance applicable to this aspect of postnatal care?
- Are there any national or international guidelines for postnatal care?
- Are there any legal issues underpinning this aspect of postnatal care?

Team working

Whilst midwives are the experts in low-risk postnatal care, they remain reliant on a number of other workers to provide a comprehensive, safe service. Midwives work as part of a team of professional and support staff who each bring particular skills and perspectives to the care of women and their families. The NMC Code requires registrants to 'keep colleagues informed when you are sharing care with others' and 'work with colleagues to monitor the quality of your work and maintain the safety of those in your care' (2008:03). It also states:

- You must work cooperatively within teams and respect the skills, expertise and contributions of your colleagues.
- You must be willing to share your skills and experience for the benefit of your colleagues.
- You must consult and take advice from colleagues when appropriate.
- You must treat your colleagues fairly and without discrimination. (NMC 2008:03)

The midwives rules and standards also requires midwives to refer any woman or baby whose condition deviates from normal to an appropriate health professional (NMC 2004:16).

Questions that need to be addressed to ensure that the woman's care makes appropriate use of the multi-professional team include:

- Does this aspect of postnatal care fall within my current role?
- Have I acknowledged the limitations of my professional knowledge?
- Who else will need to be involved in the provision of this care?
- Where is the most appropriate place to document this aspect of postnatal care?
- Who will I involve if her observations are outside normal parameters?
- How can I facilitate effective team working with this woman?
- Will another person be required to assist with this aspect of postnatal care?
- When will they be available and how can I access them?

Effective communication

Providing woman-centred care to women during the postnatal period requires midwives to engage and communicate effectively with them. It is essential that the midwife is aware of the cues she is giving to the woman during the care she provides. Time is often pressured in midwifery both in the community and hospital setting but it is important to convey to the woman that she is the focus of your attention. Taking time to explain what you are going to do and why is crucial if she is going to trust that you will always act in her best interest.

Questions that need to be addressed throughout postnatal care include:

- What opportunities are there for the woman to convey her hopes and fears in the postnatal period?
- How can the midwife facilitate meaningful discussion about her choices for care?
- What information needs to be given in order for the woman to choose whether this is the right decision for her?
- How can the partner be effectively involved in supporting the woman in the postnatal period?
- Has she given consent for me to give this aspect of care?
- Does the woman understand what the care entails?
- In what ways could the information about this aspect of care be given?
- What should be said during the care?
- What should be observed in the woman's behaviour during the care?
- What should be communicated to the woman after the care?
- How and where should recording of the care and its effectiveness be made?

Clinical dexterity

Midwives providing postnatal care need to exercise a range of skills in order to provide choice for women. They need to be able to employ competent technical knowledge when supporting a woman who is having difficulty breastfeeding as well as using effective supportive and communication skills. Midwives need to apply their experience and wisdom to facilitate successful adaptation to parenthood and have the confidence to encourage women to try alternative strategies when appropriate. The midwife continues to learn new skills throughout her working life and is accountable for maintaining and developing her practice as new ways of working are introduced (NMC 2008:04).

Questions that need to be addressed to ensure that the woman's care is provided with clinical dexterity include:

- How has postnatal care changed since I first qualified as a midwife?
- Can I provide this care in other ways?
- How has my previous experience influenced how I approach this aspect of care today?
- How can I be sure I am carrying this out correctly?
- Are there opportunities for practising this skill elsewhere?
- Who can I observe to explore alternative ways of doing this?

Models of care

One of the key policy recommendations is that women should have choice about where they receive their postnatal care (Department of Health 2007). In order to facilitate this, midwives must work in many settings and in a range of maternity care systems. For example, midwives work in primary care, providing postnatal care in women's homes, at drop-in clinics within general practitioner (GP) surgeries or in local children's centres. Midwives can also work independently providing holistic client-centred care, or within a large tertiary centre providing care for women with specific postnatal health needs. The models of care can be influential in determining the care that a woman may receive, from whom and when. Midwives need to consider the most appropriate ways that care can be delivered so that they can influence future development in the best interests of women and their families.

Questions that need to be addressed to ensure that the impact of the way that care is provided is acknowledged include:

- How long has care been provided in this way?
- How is the maternity service organized?
- Which professional groups are involved in the provision of this service?
- How is this procedure/care influenced by the model of care provided?
- How does this model of care impact on the carers?
- How does this model of care impact on the woman and her family?
- Is this the best way to provide care from a professional point of view?

Safe environment

Midwives providing postnatal care need to ensure that the environment in which they work supports safe and effective working practices and protects the woman and her family from harm. The NMC Code states that 'you must have the skills and knowledge for safe and effective practice when working without direct supervision' (NMC 2008:04). The midwife must ensure that the care she gives does not compromise the safety of women and their families. She must therefore create and maintain a safe working environment at all times, whether in a woman's home, children's centre or in a hospital service.

Questions that need to be addressed to ensure that the woman's care is provided in a safe environment include:

- Can the woman be assured that her confidentiality will be maintained?
- Does the woman understand the implications of giving her consent to this procedure?
- Are there facilities to ensure that her privacy and dignity are maintained?
- Is there somewhere to wash hands?
- Is there an appropriate place to dispose of waste?
- Is the equipment appropriately maintained and free from contamination?
- Is the space adequate to allow ease of movement around the woman without invading her personal space?
- What are the risks involved in this procedure/care and how have they been addressed?
- Are there any risks to the person undertaking this procedure/care?
- Is this environment safe for others who might come into the room?

Promotes health

Providing postnatal care for women and their families presents a unique opportunity to influence the health and wellbeing of the public. Midwives must capitalize on their contacts with women to help them achieve a positive adaptation to parenthood and promote lifestyle choices that will benefit women, babies and families in the future.

Questions that need to be addressed to ensure that the woman's care promotes health include:

- Is this procedure/care going to help her or harm her or her baby in any way?
- What are the opportunities to use this procedure to educate her/her family on healthy behaviours?
- What resources can women and families access to help them make healthy lifestyle choices?
- Has enough time been allocated to this aspect of care to make the most of the opportunities to promote healthy living?

- Who else should I involve to ensure that the woman and her family get the best possible advice in this situation?

The book begins with a chapter focusing on the principles and practice of postnatal care. The subsequent chapters use the jigsaw model to explore scenarios from practice, focusing on the role of the midwife in the various aspects of postnatal care. Thus the reader is provided with a structure with which to reflect on her care and that of the multi-professional team in which she works. Each chapter includes a range of activities designed to enable the midwife to contextualize the information within her own practice, applying her continually developing knowledge to her own circumstances. The chapters are written so that they can be accessed without having read the previous ones, although we hope you will find the whole book relevant and thought provoking.
Enjoy!

References

Department of Health: *Changing childbirth: Report of the Expert Maternity Group Pt. II, Report of the Expert Maternity Group Pt.1.* London, 1993, Department of Health.

Department of Health: *National Service Framework for children, young people and maternity services. Standard 11,* 2004, Maternity Services.

Department of Health: *Maternity matters: choice, access and continuity of care in a safe service,* London, 2007, Department of Health.

National Institute for Health and Clinical Excellence (NICE): *Routine postnatal care of women and their babies. NICE clinical guideline 37,* London, 2006, NICE.

Nursing and Midwifery Council (NMC): *Midwives rules and standards,* London, 2004, NMC.

Nursing and Midwifery Council (NMC): *The Code. Standards of conduct, performance and ethics for nurses and midwives*, London, 2008, NMC.

Nursing and Midwifery Council (NMC): *Standards for pre-registration midwifery education*, London, 2009, NMC.

Wickham S: Feminism and ways of knowing. In Stewart M, editor: *Pregnancy, birth and maternity care: feminist perspectives*, Oxford, 2004, Books for Midwives, pp 157–168.

Chapter 2

Postnatal care: principles and practice

Trigger scenario

Annie wakes with a start. Her baby is crying. A little unsure, and conscious of the other women in the ward, she gets out of bed and takes him out of the cot. She remembers how the midwife had soothed him the night before and gently rocks him and tells him who is coming to see him that day. He quietens and opens his eyes.

Introduction

The face of postnatal care is gradually changing, although this evolution has been slower in some maternity units than in others. There is more emphasis on assessing the individual needs of women rather than on applying a standard protocol to all women during every postnatal examination. However, each student midwife will need to work within locally developed guidelines and will learn 'how things are done here' from the mentorship she has and the observations she makes. This chapter outlines the underlying principles and basic content of the postnatal examination, which can be adapted to meet the individual needs of women and their babies.

What is the postnatal period?

This period has, until recently, been very strictly defined as not less than 10 days, or more than 28 days, after the end of labour (United Kingdom Central Council (UKCC) 1998). However, it has since been acknowledged that the public health role of the midwife should be further developed (Department of Health 1999), and proposals for an extension of the midwife's role within women's health were further outlined in the 'Midwifery Action Plan' (Department of Health 2001).

This concept has been reflected in the Midwives Rules and Standards (NMC 2004), which state that the 'postnatal period' is:

...the period after the end of labour during which the attendance of a midwife upon a woman and baby is required, being not less than 10 days and for such longer period as the midwife considers necessary.

(NMC 2004:07)

In practice, however, the number and content of postnatal examinations varies between individual midwives and National Health Service (NHS) Trusts. Capacity to extend postnatal visiting beyond 28 days (or even 10 days in some areas) is dependent on sufficient midwifery staffing levels and supportive evidence-based guidelines.

Postnatal care

Access to care

In the government policy document *Maternity matters* (Department of Health 2007), as part of the national choice guarantees, it was stated that when women leave hospital they should have a choice regarding where they access postnatal care. It was recommended that these choices should include in their own home or via a community service, such as in a Sure Start children's centre (Department of Health 2007:13). Some community midwives offer 'drop-in' sessions for postnatal mothers whilst others continue to provide the majority of care in the woman's home. Greater flexibility

and widening access to care is also an objective of postnatal care in other developed countries (Declercq et al 2008, McLachlan et al 2008).

What does postnatal care include?

The Midwives Rules and Standards (NMC 2004) include the 'Activities of a midwife', an extract from The European Union Second Midwifery Directive, Article 4. These activities are those that midwives are entitled to pursue within the member states, and include:

to care for and monitor the progress of the mother in the postnatal period and to give all necessary advice to the woman on infant care to enable her to ensure the optimum progress of the new born infant

(NMC 2004:37)

A key aspect of this statement is that the midwife should care for the mother. This is an essential underlying facet of midwifery practice. The woman should feel that the midwives have her best interests at heart. She needs to be listened to and heard, safe in the understanding that her values and beliefs as an individual will be honoured wherever possible. Her unique needs should be carefully assessed and her care planned to address them specifically. For example, if a midwife was caring for a woman who had symphysis pubis dysfunction (SPD), and asked her to walk down to the dining room for her meal, this could convey to the woman that she had not taken the time to find out about her individual circumstances.

It would have been much more caring if the midwife had introduced herself and acknowledged that she was aware of her SPD and that she would bring her meals to her bedside.

While most midwives will care about the women they look after, not all will demonstrate this. To ask a woman who had an episiotomy if she has any stitches, or a primiparous woman if she has breastfed before, could leave her feeling like one of many – to be processed rather than cared for.

Another element of the activity quoted is that it advocates that the midwife should provide advice to the woman to enable her to undertake her mothering role. She can do this in a number of ways. For example, the midwife who talks to the baby while undressing it acts as a role model to the woman. She demonstrates that this is appropriate behaviour, and can encourage her to do the same by informing her that the baby will probably already recognize her voice and pay particular attention to it (Damstra-Wijmenga 1991). The midwife can also praise the woman as she learns and masters her new role. Just as the student midwife needs feedback from her mentor that she is performing well, so does the new mother. We all recognize the boost that is felt when someone tells you that you did something really well. New parents also need a boost to their confidence, and this will help them develop new skills (Cronk & Flint 1989).

Giving advice and providing care for women should be based on an assessment of need. This applies to all women irrespective of parity. Rather than giving 'one size fits all' advice, which is inappropriate and rather tedious, it is more pertinent to find out what the woman already knows about a particular issue. This enables you to tailor your advice to fill the gaps in her knowledge or understanding and also, importantly, to correct misinformation.

Assumptions should not be made about the level of a woman's knowledge or her desire to receive information. A well-educated woman may need reminding not to leave her baby unattended on the bed, and a childminder may not be aware of the latest advice regarding cot death prevention. Where possible, verbal information should be supplemented by another means of reinforcement, such as written guidance or a practical demonstration. Every care should be taken to provide consistent information; conflicting advice was highlighted as a source of distress to women by the Audit Commission survey (1998). A decade later, in a subsequent survey (Commission for Healthcare Audit and Inspection 2007), lack of information remains an issue for postnatal women with only 58% saying that they always had the information and explanations they needed after the baby's birth (op cit: 14).

Quality of care

In an exploratory study of what constitutes quality in maternity care (Proctor 1998), women focused on the need for information and help to develop mothering confidence during the postnatal period. Of the midwives who were asked about what they thought were the components of good care, few identified areas of postnatal care that women had raised as important, other than support for breastfeeding. Women's perceptions of postnatal care in England have subsequently been measured in detail. In 2006 in a study of a random sample of 4800 women (Redshaw et al 2007), new mothers were more critical of the staff who cared for them than at any other time throughout their pregnancy and birth. Poor communication by one or more members of staff was an issue for 16% women and 22% reported that they had not always been treated with respect. Only 53% of the women who responded to the survey felt that they received individualized care.

Quality of postnatal care in hospital is related to staffing levels and this problem is not unique to the United Kingdom. In an Australian study (Forster et al 2006) significant issues highlighted as a result of low staffing levels included: poor staff/client ratios; inappropriate staff skill mix; high dependency of clients; labour wards taking priority and the use of agency staff. These issues require further exploration so that appropriate workable solutions can be agreed to address the impact of this deficit.

Cultural differences

Within each culture there are specific practices in relation to postnatal activity and behaviour. It is incumbent on any midwife working in a culturally diverse area to find out about the specific postnatal norms for the women she cares for. However, it is important not to make assumptions. Belonging to a particular religion or race does not necessarily mean that an individual woman will practise its doctrine to the letter. Do not be afraid to ask a woman about how her faith or ethnicity impacts on her postnatal activity; she is likely to value the interest you have taken in her own particular circumstances.

The postnatal examination

The postnatal examination involves assessment of the woman's emotional and physical wellbeing and includes evaluation of the baby's health and behaviour. It is usually performed daily in the first few days after the birth, although this pattern will vary according to need. As the woman becomes more confident and recovers from the birth, the midwife will space out the examinations, in consultation with her. For the midwife to undertake this aspect of her role, she therefore needs a clear understanding of what is normal postnatal recovery and expected neonatal behaviour. The emphasis is on confirming normality and providing the woman with feedback about her own progress. The woman should be given sufficient information to enable her to identify for herself if her health gives cause for concern.

Box 2.1 provides a summary of the possible components of a postnatal examination for the woman. On occasions it will be important to

Box 2.1 Components of the postnatal examination

- Give the woman an approximate time for when you will be available to undertake her postnatal examination

Rationale To enable the woman to plan her time accordingly – e.g. take a shower

- Inform the woman that you are ready to undertake her examination; ask her if she needs to pass urine

Rationale To provide her with the opportunity to empty her bladder

- Read her notes

Rationale To appreciate her birth experience; to identify any issues requiring special attention; to evaluate any previous care/advice

- Draw the curtains around her bed or find a place where there will not be any interruptions

Rationale To maintain her privacy and dignity, affording her the opportunity to disclose personal information

- Wash hands

Rationale To reduce the risk of cross-infection

- Seated at eye level with her, ask her how she is feeling, sleeping and eating

Rationale To assess emotional wellbeing. Sitting conveys that you are prepared to stay and listen

- Ask her how her breasts feel. Inform her how to examine her breasts and what to do if she notices any red areas or lumps

Rationale To assess if breasts are comfortable, and encourage involvement in her own postnatal recovery

- If breastfeeding, ask how her nipples feel during and after feeds

Rationale To ensure correct positioning

- Ask the woman about her blood loss. Advise her what to do if she passes any clots, or if her loss becomes heavier or offensive smelling. Advise her what to do if her abdomen becomes tender. Undertake temperature and pulse and gentle abdominal palpation if infection suspected

Rationale To assess if lochia is within normal parameters; to identify infection

- Ask the woman how she is finding passing urine since the birth. Inform her what to do if she has any frequency or pain. Encourage pelvic floor exercises

Rationale To assess her bladder function and tone and involve her in her own recovery

- Ask the woman about her bowel habits. If she has haemorrhoids, ask her how she is managing them. Offer dietary advice

Rationale To assess if bowel function has returned, and to offer advice and support

- Observe legs. Offer advice regarding oedema if present and encourage leg exercises. Advise her what to do if she has pain in her calves

Rationale To assess leg comfort, and encourage the woman to take action to help prevent deep vein thrombosis (DVT)

- Ask the woman about perineal pain or discomfort (examine if affirmative)

Rationale To assess that wounds, swelling, bruising and/or abrasions are clean and healing

continued

Box 2.1 Continued

- Ask the woman if she is doing any postnatal exercises and explain their importance

Rationale To encourage her to undertake postnatal exercises. To provide opportunity to demonstrate exercises, if appropriate

- Ask the woman if she has any concerns or questions

Rationale To provide the opportunity for unresolved concerns to be addressed

- Wash hands

Rationale To minimize the risk of cross-infection

- Complete documentation

Rationale To communicate findings and advice given to the woman

---

undertake most or all of these steps, but as the woman recovers from the birth the examination should become less clinical and focus more on her wellbeing. A general principle is that observations should be continued until they maintain a normal result, unless underlying disease is suspected and a more conservative approach is required. Verbal consent from the woman must be gained before any aspect of the examination is undertaken on either herself or her baby. All abnormal findings observed by a student midwife should be documented and reported to a practising midwife.

Wellbeing

The midwife assesses the woman's emotional wellbeing by observing her body language and general activity. Does she appear well rested and relaxed? Is she participating in her usual daily activities, taking care with her hygiene and communicating with those around her? The midwife also uses open-ended questions to enable the

woman to articulate how she is feeling and to express any concerns. In order to facilitate this process, however, the midwife needs to convey that she has time to listen and respond to any issues that are raised. This may be difficult during a busy working day, but is an investment in helping to prevent minor concerns from becoming a source of unnecessary anguish. Women should be asked at every postnatal examination about their mood and support networks (NICE 2006). Chapter 8 focuses on maternal postnatal wellbeing in further detail.

Activity

List the possible causes of an elevated maternal temperature during the puerperium.

Consider in what circumstances it would be prudent to take regular measurements of temperature and pulse.

Observations

The woman's temperature, pulse and blood pressure are recorded immediately after the birth (NICE 2007) and usually again an hour later to confirm that they remain within normal limits. Women who have had an elevated blood pressure in the absence of other symptoms of pre-eclampsia should have their blood pressure repeated within 4 hours (NICE 2007). If other signs are present, her condition should be investigated with urgency. Women on anti-hypertensive medication should also have regular blood pressure measurements taken. Women should be advised regarding the symptoms of pre-eclampsia and when to seek medical care.

In the absense of any cause to suspect infection, routine temperature measurement is not indicated (NICE 2006) as it is unlikely to prevent morbidity. Takahashi (1998), in an evaluation of routine maternal temperature measurement, concluded that as a screening tool it had limited usefulness, having poor sensitivity and specificity. How often observations of temperature and pulse continue depends on local policy.

Breasts

The woman should be asked how her breasts feel and advised about what to expect in the following days and weeks. It is not necessary to inspect the breasts unless there is a concern raised. For example, if – when asked – the woman is unable to confirm that there are no red areas or lumps then it would be appropriate to observe them, with consent, and show her how to make sure all is well.

Activity

Consider what action you would take if a woman had a pink area on her breast.

Think about how you would respond if a woman detected a lump in her breast.

Note down the advice you would give a woman who was breastfeeding and complaining of sore nipples.

Uterine involution

The term 'uterine involution' refers to the return of the uterus to a pelvic organ (Bick et al 2008). Palpating the height of the uterine fundus has traditionally been considered a fundamental aspect of the postnatal examination: 'the uterine fundus should be palpated each postnatal day to exclude any complication' (Hynes 1999:598). However, the value of this procedure has since been questioned (Montgomery & Alexander 1994). Not only does the rate of uterine involution vary between individual women (Cluett et al 1997) but there are differences between the same and different midwives estimation of the symphysis–fundal height (Cluett et al 1995). In a study exploring postnatal blood loss (BLiPP) Marchant et al (2000) found considerable variation in the way that involution is measured (by finger breadths or measurement) and in the way that findings are documented. Although the research did not advocate one method of measurement over another, the authors concluded that a consistent approach should be adopted in order to detect potential morbidity.

Routine estimation of fundal height is no longer advocated (NICE 2006). However, when infection is suspected, it can provide useful information and a baseline for further evaluation. Assessment of uterine fundal height is undertaken by external abdominal palpation. The midwife uses her non-dominant hand and, starting at the umbilicus, uses the pads of her middle three fingers gently to locate the fundus. She works down the abdomen, finger breadth by finger breadth, until she meets the firm resistance of the involuting uterus. The uterus should be central and non-tender and be diminishing in size on successive examinations. Sub-involution (delayed return of the uterus to its pre-pregnant size) could be caused by infection or retained products of conception and would require referral to a doctor.

Activity

Identify the process by which the uterus resumes its pre-pregnancy size.

List factors which could cause the fundal height to be higher than expected.

Find out what is meant by the term 'anthropometry'.

Make sure you know what 'after pains' are.

Blood loss

The blood that is lost following childbirth is called lochia. The amount of lochia, its colour and duration vary between individual women. In a large prospective study, Marchant et al (1999) found that the average duration was 21 days with a range of 10–42 days. Women need to be aware of this large variation and to seek advice if their lochia becomes offensive in odour or suddenly increases in amount.

Bladder

Occasionally, bladder tone is reduced following the birth and the woman may need support and information. She should be advised to empty her bladder regularly and to drink freely, according to her thirst. Pelvic floor exercises should be encouraged. If the woman is experiencing incontinence (other than when she coughs or sneezes), or has pain on micturition, a specimen of urine should be sent to the laboratory to exclude infection, and medical advice sought.

Bowels

Women often worry about opening their bowels after childbirth, particularly if they have stitches. They may value advice about which foods are high in fibre and ensuring an adequate fluid intake. A woman may find it useful to hold a folded sanitary pad over her stitches and apply pressure over them when she attempts to go to the toilet for the first time after giving birth.

Legs

The woman's legs should be observed for any calf swelling, pain or inflammation. If there is a question or uncertainty regarding a difference in size between the calves, then a tape measure should be used to measure the widest circumference. Ankle and/or pre-tibial oedema sometimes occurs following the birth. This is normal, and the woman should be encouraged to perform regular ankle rotation exercises and to elevate her feet while resting. Flexing the leg at the knee and dorsiflexing the ankle (Homan's sign) is not advocated as a method for detecting thromboembolism (Urbano 2001).

Perineum

The woman should be asked about her perineum at each visit and the midwife should assess it if she complains of pain or odour (NICE 2006). The perineum is most easily examined if the woman is lying down, rolls away from you on to her side and bends her knees slightly. Wearing gloves, the uppermost buttock can be lifted gently to reveal the perineal area. The midwife should provide feedback to the woman about what she observes – for example, that her stitches are clean and healing well and that the swelling has gone. If she has haemorrhoids, she will benefit from a high-fibre diet and a prescription for some anti-inflammatory analgesic cream. The perineum can be a source of discomfort; the woman should be offered regular analgesia.

Postnatal exercises

These should be encouraged and demonstrated if necessary. Women often feel frustrated with their post-pregnancy figure and need reassurance that they can regain or even improve on their physical fitness after the birth. Only gentle exercise should be attempted in the first few weeks due to the lingering effects of progesterone on the ligaments.

The baby examination

The baby is examined daily by the midwife in the first few days of life. The order in which the woman and the baby are examined depends on the circumstances, including who is on hand to help with the baby and whether the baby is hungry and demanding a feed. The guiding principle should be: avoid disturbing a baby until or unless there is someone who can comfort him/her afterwards. If the baby is settled at the beginning of the examination, then the woman should be examined first, so that she will be available to attend to her baby after his/her examination. However, if the baby is unsettled at the beginning of the examination, then it would be prudent to look at the baby first and then settle the baby, as the woman is unlikely to feel relaxed and ask questions if her baby is crying in the background.

It is important to ask the woman's permission to disturb her baby for its examination as she may have only just settled him/her after a long and difficult night. It may be possible to postpone the examination or to talk through it, rather than wake the baby. Before the baby is disturbed, a warm place should be identified where he/she can be unwrapped in full view of the mother. If at home, this might be on a changing mat on the floor, with a soft sheet or towel placed over the plastic. Experienced midwives often check the baby on their knee. This should only be attempted once confidence in handling the newborn has been gained. A protective, waterproof apron should be worn to avoid seepage of unexpected bodily fluids through to your clothes. A firm hand should always have hold of the baby, and s/he should always be turned towards you rather than away when looking at his/her back. The baby on your knee should lie across your legs rather than with his/her feet in your stomach. Even very young babies can push against you and move backwards.

Box 2.2 provides a summary of components of a well baby examination.

Fontanelles

The anterior fontanelle should be flat while the baby is quiet, although in a crying baby with little hair it may be seen to bulge (Baston & Durward 2001).

Umbilicus

Parents are sometimes reluctant to handle the cord stump, and require reassurance that it does not hurt the baby. The cord separates from the navel by a process of dry gangrene. Current practice advocates that the cord is cleaned with water at nappy changes (NICE 2006) as the application of antibiotic powder and alcohol swabs do not reduce the risk of infection (Capurro 2004). The cord stump will dry out and separate, usually within 10 days. The skin around the navel should not be red or inflamed (Johnson & Taylor 2006).

Skin integrity

A large part of the baby examination involves exploring the baby's skin to ensure that the skin is healthy and intact. As the baby has many skin folds – for example, in the crease of the neck or in the axilla – it is important that they are kept clean and dry to avoid infection. The baby's nails should be examined to ensure that paranikia are not developing, and that there are no pieces of nail that could scratch the baby's skin.

Feeding

The woman should be asked how feeding is going. If she is breastfeeding, she may ask how often or for how long the baby should feed. Emphasis should be on helping her to feel confident that the baby is getting enough milk because her breasts soften after a feed, the baby settles and has plenty of wet and soiled nappies. The term baby should be demand-fed. For a baby fed on artificial milk this will average approximately 150–180 ml/kg/day (Roberton 1996).

Box 2.2 The baby examination

- Ask the woman's permission to examine her baby and explain what you are going to do

Rationale To ensure that she consents to her baby being disturbed

- Prepare a safe, warm place to examine the baby, with nappy-changing equipment at hand

Rationale To provide a setting where the baby can be observed by its mother.

- Wash and dry hands

Rationale To warm them and reduce the risk of cross-infection

- Place the baby on a flat surface and observe activity and tone

Rationale To assess moving all its limbs equally and has flexed tone

- Examine fontanelles, scalp, behind ears and crease of neck

Rationale To assess hydration and skin integrity

- Observe eyes

Rationale To assess that both eyes are clear from infection

- With dominant thumb on baby's chin, open his/her mouth and inspect tongue

Rationale To assess that the tongue is clear from infection

- Examine hands and fingers

Rationale To assess skin integrity and that nails are short

- Take off clothes (leave nappy on). Lift each arm up and examine axilla

Rationale To assess skin integrity and muscle tone

- Examine legs and feet

Rationale To assess skin integrity and muscle tone

- Turn baby over, supported on your non-dominant hand

Rationale To assess skin integrity. and examine back

- Examine umbilicus

Rationale To assess that cord stump is drying; to assess skin integrity

- Remove nappy, clean skin and re-dress baby

Rationale To assess skin integrity; to keep baby warm

- Ask the woman about the number of wet nappies the baby has each day

Rationale To assess adequate hydration and bladder function

- Ask the woman about the frequency of baby's bowel motions and colour and consistency of the stools

Rationale To assess that the baby is well hydrated and receiving adequate milk intake

- Hand baby back to mother

Rationale To enable baby to be comforted and to allow mother–infant interaction to be observed

- Wash hands

Rationale To minimize the risk of cross-infection

- Ask the woman about baby's feeding pattern

Rationale To ensure baby is demanding feeds

- Complete documentation

Rationale To communicate findings and advice to woman and colleagues

After two to three days, the baby's stools change from black meconium to yellow/brown. A breastfed baby passes unformed stools, sometimes at every feed, whereas the baby fed on artificial milk passes formed stools, just once or twice a day. The baby should pass pale urine, usually at every feed. For further information about supporting a woman to feed her baby, see Chapter 10.

Conclusion

The midwife makes a detailed assessment of both the woman and her baby's progress regularly in the first few days after the birth. As they grow in confidence, midwifery input can be gradually withdrawn to enable the new parents to further develop their parenting skills. Parents will face times when they need to assess if their baby's behaviour is within normal limits. The role of the midwife is to equip them with the necessary skills and confidence to know when their baby is well and thriving or when to seek professional help.

Resources

Maternity Matters. Choice, access and continuity of care in a safe service. http://www.dh.gov.uk/en/Publicationsandstatistics/Publications/PublicationsPolicyAndGuidance/DH_073312.

NICE: Intrapartum care guidelines. http://www.nice.org.uk/nicemedia/pdf/IPCNICEGuidance.pdf.

NICE: Postnatal care guidelines. http://www.nice.org.uk/nicemedia/pdf/CG37NICEguideline.pdf.

Recorded delivery: a national survey of women's experience of maternity care 2006. http://www.npeu.ox.ac.uk/downloads/maternitysurveys/maternity-survey-report.pdf.

Saving mothers' lives. Key recommendations for midwives: http://www.cemach.org.uk/getattachment/7654804a-9442-4a30-8857-4c2ec4391ae3/Saving-Mothers'-Lives-2003-2005_MidwifSumm.aspx.

Women's experience of maternity care in the NHS in England. http://www.healthcarecommission.org.uk/_db/_documents/Maternity_services_survey_report.pdf.

References

Audit Commission: *First class delivery. A national survey of women's views of maternity care*, London, 1998, Audit Commission.

Baston H, Durward H: *Examination of the newborn. A practical guide*, London, 2001, Routledge.

Bick D, MacArthur C, Knowles H, et al: *Postnatal care: evidence and guidelines for management,* ed 2, Edinburgh, 2008, Churchill Livingstone.

Capurro H: Routine topical umbilical cord care at birth: RHL commentary. *The WHO Reproductive Health Library, No 9.* Oxford, 2004, Update Software Ltd. Online. Available www.rhlibrary.com.

Cluett E, Alexander J, Pickering R: Is measuring the symphysis–fundal distance worthwhile? *Midwifery* 11(4):174–183, 1995.

Cluett E, Alexander J, Pickering R: What is the normal pattern of uterine involution? An investigation of postpartum uterine involution measured by the distance between the symphysis pubis and the uterine fundus using a tape measure, *Midwifery* 13(1):9–16, 1997.

Commission for Healthcare Audit and Inspection: *Women's experiences of maternity care in the NHS in England,* London, 2007, Healthcare Commission.

Cronk M, Flint C: *Community midwifery: a practical guide,* Oxford, 1989, Heinemann Nursing.

Damstra-Wijmenga S: The memory of the newborn baby, *Midwives' Chronicle* 104(1238):66–69, 1991.

Declercq E, Sakala C, Corry MP, et al: *New mothers speak out. National survey results highlight women's postpartum experiences,* New York, 2008, Childbirth Connections.

Department of Health: *Making a difference: strengthening the nursing, midwifery and health visiting contribution to health and health care,* London, 1999, Department of Health.

Department of Health: *Making a difference: the nursing, midwifery and health visiting contribution. The Midwifery Action Plan,* London, 2001, Department of Health.

Department of Health: *Maternity matters: choice, access and continuity of care in a safe service,* London, 2007, Department of Health.

Forster D, Mclachlan H, Yelland J, et al: Staffing in postnatal units: is it inadequate for the provision of quality care? Staff perspectives from a state wide review of psotnatal care in Victoria, Australia, *BMC Health Service Research* 4(6):83, 2006.

Hynes L: Physiology, complications and management of the puerperium. In Bennett V, Brown L, editors: *Myles' text book for midwives,* ed 13, Edinburgh, 1999, Churchill Livingstone.

Johnson R, Taylor W: *Skills for midwifery practice,* ed 2, Edinburgh, 2006, Harcourt Health Sciences.

Marchant S, Alexander J, Garcia J, et al: A survey of women's experiences of vaginal loss from 24 hours to three months after childbirth (the BLIPP study), *Midwifery* 15(2):72–81, 1999.

Marchant S, Alexander J, Garcia J: How does it feel to you? Uterine palpation and lochial loss as guides to postnatal "recovery". 2 – The BLiPP study (blood loss in the postnatal period), *The Practising Midwife* 3(7):31–33, 2000.

McLachlan HL, Forster DA, Davey MA, et al: *COSMOS: Comparing standard maternity care with one-to-one midwifery support: a randomised controlled trial*, 2008, Biomed Central, Pregnancy and Childbirth. Online. Available http://www.biomedcentral.com/1471-2393/8/35, January 16, 2009.

Montgomery E, Alexander J: Assessing postnatal uterine involution: a review and a challenge, *Midwifery* 10(2): 73–76, 1994.

National Institute for Health and Clinical Excellence (NICE): *Routine postnatal care of women and their babies*, London, 2006, NICE.

National Insitute for Health and Clinical Excellence (NICE): *Intrapartum care. Care of healthy women and their babies during childbirth. NICE clinical guideline 55*, London, 2007, NICE.

Nursing and Midwifery Council (NMC): *Midwives Rules and Standards*, London, 2004, NMC.

Proctor S: What determines quality in maternity care? Comparing the perceptions of childbearing women and midwives, *Birth* 25(2):85–93, 1998.

Redshaw M, Rowe R, Hockley C, et al: *Recorded delivery: a national survey of women's experience of maternity care*, Oxford, 2007, National Perinatal Epidemiology Unit.

Roberton N: *A manual of normal neonatal care*, London, 1996, Arnold.

Takahashi H: Evaluating routine postnatal maternal temperature check, *British Journal of Midwifery* 6(3):139–143, 1998.

United Kingdom Central Council (UKCC): *Midwives Rules and Code of Practice*, London, 1998, UKCC.

Urbano F: Homans' sign in the diagnosis of deep venous thrombosis, *Hospital Physician* 37(3):22–24, 2001.

Chapter 3

Care of the baby at birth

Trigger scenario

Teresa had her legs in stirrups and a doctor sitting between them. Her partner had gone out of the room to speak to his parents. The midwife and student had their backs to her, leaning over the plastic crib that held her baby. They were talking intently but Teresa could not hear what they were saying. 'Is he alright?' she asked.

Introduction

The midwife who cares for a woman in labour has a dual responsibility. She endeavours to ensure that the needs of the woman and her partner are met while keeping a careful watch on the health of the unborn baby. Once the baby is born, the need to assess the baby's wellbeing continues as it makes the transition to extra-uterine life. This chapter describes the care of the baby in the immediate perinatal period, how its adaptation to the outside world is assessed, and how it is examined by the midwife. The recommendations of the National Institute for Health and Clinical Excellence (NICE 2007) are summarized in Box 3.1.

Individualized care

Before the baby is born, the woman should be asked about her wishes for the birth. For example, she may wish to hold her baby as soon as the trunk emerges and bring it towards the warmth of her body. Alternatively, she might prefer that the baby is dried off and wrapped up before she holds it. It should not be assumed that a woman who has not voiced any preference does not have one. Some women do not feel able to ask for anything 'out of the ordinary' and may regret not having had the opportunity to be more involved. It is attention to the details of a woman's birth that makes her feel treated as an individual and enables her to look back favourably on her experience and care. Care should

> **Box 3.1** Care of the well baby at birth (Source: NICE 2007)
>
> - Record the Apgar score at 1 and 5 minutes
> - Encourage skin-to-skin contact as soon as possible after birth
> - Dry baby and cover with warm dry blanket, while maintaining skin-to-skin contact
> - Avoid separating the mother and baby during the first hour
> - Encourage breastfeeding as soon as possible or within the first hour
> - Record head circumference, temperature and weight after the first hour
> - Conduct an initial examination of the baby to detect major physical abnormality and identify problems that may require referral to another professional
> - Gain consent prior to examination or treatment of the baby
> - Conduct examinations in the presence or knowledge of the parents.

be tailored to her particular needs and wishes, taking into account her views, values and cultural beliefs (NICE 2006).

Care of the baby

Maintaining baby's temperature

Once the baby is born, the time should be noted and the woman should receive her baby according to her wishes. The priority is to keep the baby warm: as it transfers from body temperature to room temperature it will use up vital energy to keep warm. The parents can be encouraged to dry the baby with a warm towel, which should then be discarded and replaced with another warm, dry towel. Keeping the baby close to the mother is the most effective means of maintaining and restoring a baby's body temperature (Christensson et al 1998, Walters et al 2007). Babies can lose a lot of heat from their heads, and it should remain covered until it is ascertained that the

baby is maintaining a temperature above 36.5°C. In a randomized controlled trial comparing skin-to-skin contact after birth with routine care (drying and wrapping the baby) babies who received skin-to-skin contact had significantly higher temperatures than babies in the control group (Carfoot et al 2005). Skin-to-skin contact has also been found to have additional benefits. In a systematic review of early skin-to-skin contact between the mother and baby (at birth or within 24 hours), reviewers found a positive impact on breastfeeding duration, respiration stability, mother–infant attachement and infant crying (Moore et al 2007).

Activity

Consider how a baby could potentially lose heat through: evaporation, conduction, convection and radiation.

List ways in which the midwife can reduce the risk of hypothermia in the neonate.

Clamping and cutting the cord

Prior to separating the baby from the umbilical cord, the midwife should obtain the woman's consent. Some women prefer for the cord to have stopped pulsating prior to it being cut as delayed cord clamping has been shown to raise the iron status in the baby for up to 6 months (McDonald & Middleton 2008). This practice has also been associated with an increased risk of jaundice requiring phototherapy and parents should also be given this information.

Following negotiation with the midwife, some partners wish to participate in the birth by cutting the cord, and this involvement should be facilitated where appropriate. First the midwife clamps the cord approximately halfway along its length. She then squeezes a short section of cord after the clamp and applies a second clamp, leaving a blood-free section of cord that can be cut without spraying blood. Once the cord has been cut, a smaller, more secure plastic cord clamp can be attached, approximately 1 cm from the umbilicus. The excess cord can be removed, leaving 0.5 cm of cord above the clamp.

Apgar score

The Apgar score is a tool developed to assess the physical condition of the baby at birth (Apgar 1953). Five dimensions – heart rate, respiratory effort, muscle tone, response to stimuli and colour – are given a score of zero, one or two.

Thus, the maximum score is 10 (see Table 3.1). However, this is not always achieved as many babies have blue hands and feet so soon after birth. This assessment is normally undertaken at 1 minute after the birth, and again at 5 minutes. The Apgar score is repeated if the score is less than seven at 10 minutes.

There have been minor adaptations to the original score, but in essence it has been unchanged and commonly adopted (Michaelides 2004). While the Apgar is a useful tool for assessment of the neonate at birth, it does not differentiate the underlying neonatal condition. A score of five at 1 minute could be given to a baby who was not breathing, had blue extremities, grimaced when a nasal suction catheter was used, had a normal tone and a heart rate of fewer than 100 beats per minute. However, another baby who was pink, with a normal heart rate, gasped at birth yet was limp and did not respond to oral suction could also have a score of five at 1 minute (Roberton 1996). As these babies would require different treatments, any Apgar score would need to be followed with a detailed report of the baby's clinical condition.

For the majority of babies, the Apgar score can be noted while the baby is in its parents' arms. With experience, the assessment can be made adeptly without any disturbance to the parents' interaction with their baby. In a baby that is active, pink and crying, two fingers placed over the sternum should detect a rapid heart rate – and a glance at the baby's

Table 3.1 The Apgar score

Score	0	1	2
Heart rate	Absent	Fewer than 100 beats per minute	More than 100 beats per minute
Respiratory effort	Absent	Slow or irregular	Good or crying
Muscle tone	Limp	Some flexion of limbs	Active
Reflex irritability	None	Grimace	Cough or sneeze
Colour	Blue, pale	Body pink, hands/feet blue	Completely pink

hands and feet will complete the assessment. Reflex irritability refers to the baby's response to a suction catheter introduced into its nose and mouth. In the baby described above, it can be assumed that it would object to suction – hence, a formal test of this aspect of the Apgar is unnecessary.

However, in a baby who does not make respiratory effort, is pale or limp, a more formal assessment is required in an environment where the baby can be kept warm, carefully observed and given emergency resuscitation if needed.

Resuscitation equipment

In a maternity unit, the resuscitaire provides a suitable environment. This is a piece of labour ward equipment that is available for all births, although not necessarily in the birthing room. It has an overhead radiant heater, light source, suction apparatus and an oxygen supply. In some units, careful design of the birthing rooms may mean that this equipment is discreetly hidden, available for use if required. However, in some large maternity units the resuscitaire is a mobile platform that is a feature of most rooms. Whatever the setting, including the home, resuscitation equipment should always be available and checked prior to the birth, for use in the event of unexpected neonatal compromise.

Checklist for a home birth

Check the resuscitation equipment and procedure at a home birth with reference to the following list:

■ What equipment does a midwife take to a home birth?

■ Is there a heat/light source that works and a supply of warm, dry towels?

■ Is suction available, fitted with the correct catheter and in working order?

- Is an oxygen supply available, fitted with an appropriate mask and in working order?
- Is there an accessible line of communication for paediatric assistance?
- Are neonatal drugs available, checked and with means of administration?

Activity

List factors which could result in the baby making slow respiratory effort at birth.

Find out what your local guidelines recommend for the care of a baby where the liquor had been meconium stained during labour.

Naming the baby

At some time during labour, the parents are usually asked if they have chosen any names for their baby. Choosing the baby's name is a very personal affair, and the midwife should not pass judgment on what she feels is an unsuitable name. The way that the parents want a name to be spelled should also be respected. Parents often know the baby's sex and are already calling it by name. Others may still feel undecided about their baby's name, whether or not they know the sex.

As the baby must be labelled shortly after it is born, some decision needs to be agreed regarding what to put on the label. If the parents are not married, or the woman has a different surname to her husband, the mother's surname must always be used. This is so that babies can be matched with mothers in the event of a ward evacuation and this should be sensitively explained to parents. Unmarried parents should be reassured that the father's surname can be registered on the birth certificate, provided both parents attend the registrar's office.

As soon as practicable after the birth, the baby should have two labels attached, one to each leg. Before the labels are finally written, confirmation of the agreed name needs to be sought. Unit policy varies regarding whether the woman's hospital number is also included on the label. It should at least have the baby's full name and date and time of birth written in permanent ink. The parents should be shown the labels before they are secured. Care should be taken to make sure that the labels are not too tight. If the labels are too loose they could fall off. Parents need to be advised to let a midwife know if labels are lost or appear to cause any irritation.

Weighing the baby

The weight of the baby is an essential part of the information expected by relatives and friends. It is likely, therefore, that parents will want this information quite soon after the birth, although the midwife should always seek their permission. The scales should be brought close to the parents and they should be given the opportunity to get the camera ready before the baby is unwrapped. The scales should be set at zero and lined with a clean, soft paper tissue to avoid startling the baby with the cold, hard surface. The naked baby should be gently lowered into the scales, a reading (and photo) taken and then quickly wrapped and returned to the parents. The weight should be documented in grams but converted to pounds and ounces for the parents. The median weight of a full-term baby (40 weeks' gestation) in England is 3460 g (7 lb 10 oz) (The Information Centre 2007).

The first feed

All babies should be given the opportunity for close contact with their mother after the birth. For women who are going to breastfeed, this closeness can naturally evolve into suckling at the breast. In an American study of 1085 women (DiGirolamo et al 2001), a significant factor related to early cessation of breastfeeding was late initiation (more than 1 hour after the birth). The midwife needs to take her cues from the woman and her baby. The woman may wish to wait until suturing (if required) has been undertaken, as she will be able to move into a comfortable position more easily and feel more relaxed. The unique combination of circumstances at each birth necessitates that the midwife assesses each mother/infant dyad individually rather than applying a blanket rule of 'first we do this, then we do that'. The woman may prefer that suturing is delayed until she has fed the baby. However, it may be necessary to provide guidance – for example, if a perineal wound is bleeding and requires prompt suturing then it would be appropriate to recommend that suturing takes priority.

During the first hour after birth, the baby is often very alert. It is therefore important to make the most of this opportunity and encourage the baby to feed within the hour rather than trying to feed a baby who has fallen asleep. A successful first feed is a great boost to a woman's confidence in her ability to breastfeed her baby. However, if this is not possible, for whatever reason, the woman should be reassured that successful feeding can still be established. She should be helped into a comfortable position, either lying (if she has sutures or an abdominal wound) or sitting upright. The baby should be at the same level as the breast with his or her body turned towards the woman: head, neck and back almost in a straight line (Renfrew et al 2004). The baby's mouth should be at the same level as the nipple. The weight of the baby can be supported on pillows. If the woman cradles the baby in her non-dominant arm, she can use her dominant hand to support her breast and gently stroke the baby's lips with the nipple. When the baby opens his or her mouth widely, the head can be brought towards the breast. The midwife supporting this feed must make sure that she is comfortable herself, and that she quietly guides and confirms the woman's actions. There should be no need to take hold of the woman's breast or force the baby onto the nipple. Patience and presence are key to being supportive at this stage.

If the baby is going to be fed artificial milk by bottle, new parents will also require support and guidance. It is often taken for granted that the partner will feed the baby: while this might be the plan, it should not be assumed. Whoever is feeding the baby should be seated and cradle the baby close, so that eye contact can be maintained. The teat of the bottle should be brushed against the baby's lips and inserted (on top of the tongue) when the baby opens its mouth. The milk should always cover the neck of the bottle so that the baby does not suck in air, and the cap should always be replaced over the teat when not in the baby's mouth. A typical first feed is 20–40 ml of milk. Feeding is discussed in further detail in Chapter 10.

Midwife baby examination

When any necessary suturing has been completed and the woman is comfortable and able to take part, a top-to-toe examination of her baby should be undertaken by the midwife. This is separate and distinct from the 'neonatal examination' which is a clinical examination undertaken either by a midwife or neonatal nurse who has undergone further preparation and assessment in this procedure, or by a paediatrician (see Chapter 4). The check should be delayed if the baby's temperature is 36.5°C or less, and action should be taken to warm the baby – such as skin-to-skin contact with a parent, putting on a hat and use of an electric heated pad when the baby is in the cot.

Examination of the baby is part of the midwife's role (NMC 2004:37). It should be conducted with the permission of the parents and, where possible, within their sight and with their active involvement. Detection of major abnormality at birth is increasingly rare, following the use of routine detailed ultrasound scanning during pregnancy. The midwife would discuss any unusual features with the parents, describing the findings rather than making a diagnosis. Senior midwifery and medical advice should be sought only with the parents' knowledge. It would be to betray their trust for a paediatrician unexpectedly to enter the room and say, 'I hear there is a problem with her feet,' if this were the first the parents knew of any concern.

The room should be warm and draught-free, as the baby will be naked for most of the examination. A clean, dry place should be identified so that the parents have a clear view of their baby. At home, this is easy, as it can be undertaken on a towel on a double bed or carpet. In hospital, narrow delivery beds make this more difficult and it may be safest to perform the examination with the baby in the cot. If this is the case, the cot should be wheeled to the bedside.

The midwife will first wash her hands, not only as a means of reducing cross-infection, but also to warm them. Non-sterile gloves should be worn. A running commentary should be given to the parents throughout, as well as talking to the baby. Emphasis should be given to normality, for example,

'Look at her beautifully formed spine', rather than, 'I'm looking for evidence of spina bifida.' It is through understanding and recognizing what is normal that midwives can quickly detect when this is not the case (Baston & Durward 2001).

Head and neck

The face should firstly be viewed as a whole. Are all the features present and symmetrical? Before the baby is unwrapped totally, the head should be exposed and examined for lumps and abrasions. The fontanelles can then be identified. It should be explained to the parents that the anterior fontanelle, which is large and kite-shaped, will not close until the baby is about 18 months old. The posterior fontanelle is much smaller and is closed by about 6 weeks of age. Parents should be reassured that, while it would not be prudent to apply pressure to the fontanelles, gentle rubbing (such as during a hairwash) is perfectly safe. The anterior fontanelle should be neither bulging nor sunken. The suture lines between fontanelles should not exceed 1 cm and may be felt to overlap due to moulding during the birth.

The eyelids should be opened to ensure there are eyes in the sockets. The position of the ears should be noted, along with skin tags or creases. Both nostrils should be patent (open), as babies are nasal breathers.

Next, the mouth should be opened and checked for cleft palate (visualizing with a torch and a clean little finger), teeth, tongue-tie and cysts. It is usual for the baby to respond by sucking. The parents can be shown how a newborn baby will turn, when touched at the side of the mouth, towards the stimulus.

Babies have short necks, but the chin should be extended to look at the skin integrity and check movement. The clavicles can be inspected at this time, to exclude fractures.

Trunk, spine and genitalia

The midwife examines the trunk, which should be pink and have two nipples (it is common for boys or girls to have some palpable breast tissue). The cord clamp should be secure on the umbilical cord stump. The baby should be breathing regularly (quietly) with no sternal recession. The genitalia should be inspected to confirm the sex. In a boy, the testes should be palpable in the scrotum and the urethra should open at the tip of the penis. In a girl, the clitoris and vulva may appear quite large, especially in a premature baby, but should be assessed in comparison with associated structures. When the baby passes urine for the first time this should be documented.

Holding the baby over the non-dominant hand, face down (ventral suspension), the midwife then runs the index finger slowly down the baby's spine, confirming integrity of the skin, uniformity of the spine and an absence of dimples and cysts. The buttock should be parted to locate the anus, which should appear perforate, which the passage of meconium will confirm. In this position, a baby with normal tone will attempt to raise its head and legs.

Activity

Define positional talipes.
Note which features might lead you to suspect a baby had Down's syndrome and what action you would take.
Describe five reflexes present in the baby at birth.

Limbs

The baby should be observed to be moving all limbs equally. Each arm should be lifted to inspect the axilla, and then the fingers counted. When both wrists are grasped and the baby pulled up into a sitting position, the head will lag at first and then come into line before falling onto the chest. The legs should be the same lengths. It is not necessary to undertake tests to establish

hip stability during this initial check, as these will be undertaken during the clinical examination of the newborn. It has been suggested (Moore 1989) that the examination itself could lead to hip instability. The feet should be in line with the legs, and have a mobile ankle and five toes each.

Following the examination, the baby should be dressed and given back to the mother to hold close and warm up. All findings and action taken should be documented in the baby and maternal notes.

Vitamin K

The midwife's care of the new family is not complete until the issue of vitamin K has been raised and discussed as a measure to prevent haemolytic disease of the newborn. All babies are offered vitamin K at birth, however, there has been much debate over the past decade regarding the safest route of administration for this drug. Prior to 1992 in the UK, vitamin K was routinely administered via the intramuscular route. However, publication of a controversial paper (Golding et al 1992) that suggested that vitamin K given intramuscularly was associated with childhood leukaemia led many maternity units to change their policies and provide oral preparations. However, while absolute safety cannot be assured, a pooled analysis of six case-control studies (Roman et al 2002) found no link with intramuscular vitamin K and childhood leukaemia. Parents need to have access to information regarding this issue, with clear guidance regarding local policy. Verbal consent should be sought, and decisions and preparations administered should be clearly documented.

Activity

Find out what the vitamin K policy recommends where you work.
  Investigate what information is available for parents regarding vitamin K.

Reflection on trigger

Look back on the trigger scenario.

Teresa had her legs in stirrups and a doctor sitting between them. Her partner had gone out of the room to speak to his parents. The midwife and student had their backs to her, leaning over the plastic crib that held her baby. They were talking intently but Teresa could not hear what they were saying. 'Is he alright?' she asked.

Now that you are familiar with care of the baby at birth you should have insight into how the scenario relates to the evidence about this aspect of the midwife's role. The jigsaw model will now be used to explore the trigger scenario in more depth.

Effective communication

The woman's need for information and feedback does not end following the birth. She will remain sensitive to any suggestion that there might be a concern about her baby's wellbeing.

When the woman's partner is not available to act as a go-between for the woman and her carers, it is even more important that midwives include the woman in all discussions. Questions that arise from the scenario might include: How can the midwife and the student ensure that they communicate effectively with the woman? What are they discussing? Is there ever a need to discuss the baby's condition in private? Have they sought the consent of the woman before examining her baby?

Woman-centred care

Teresa is in a vulnerable position. She has her legs in stirrups and is probably having her perineum sutured. The provision of woman-centred care relies on carers concentrating on the individual needs of women and prioritizing those over their own. It might be more efficient to examine the baby while Teresa is being sutured but it deprives Teresa of attention when she needs it and excludes her from the activity.

Questions that arise from the scenario might include: As the woman's partner has left the room, who is supporting Teresa whilst she is in this undignified position? Could the examination of the baby have waited until Teresa was in a more comfortable position and able to participate in her baby's first top-to-toe examination?

Using best evidence

Midwives have a duty to provide care based on 'locally agreed evidence based standards'

(NMC 2004:18, NMC 2008:04). Despite this obligation, care is not always provided in a way that best meets the needs of the woman and her family.

Questions that arise from the scenario might include: Are there any guidelines that describe when and how the first examination of the baby takes place? If so, who was involved in their compilation? How is the implementation of evidence-based guidelines audited? What factors influence why professionals do not always adhere to guidelines?

Professional and legal issues

To provide safe and effective care midwives must work within the professional framework as determined by the Nursing and Midwifery Council. They must comply with the law and work within the terms of their employment contract (when applicable). Questions that arise from the scenario might include: Have the midwives sought and gained informed consent from Teresa before examining her baby? Did they explain the nature of the examination? In what circumstances can a midwife perform care without prior consent? Was Teresa asked if the student midwife could be involved in her care? Are the midwives working in Teresa's best interests by examining her baby out of earshot?

Team working

Midwives work as a member of a multi-professional, multi-agency team. Although they are able to provide care to a woman and her baby who are deemed 'low-risk' or making 'normal' progress, they are also required to refer any concerns to an appropriately qualified health professional who can assist in the provision of care (NMC 2004:16). Questions that arise from the scenario might include: Why is the doctor suturing Teresa's perineum? In what circumstances should this procedure be undertaken by a midwife? How does the student midwife learn to suture? If the midwives detect an abnormality in the baby during this first examination, whom should they inform first?

Clinical dexterity

Practicing clinical midwifery requires the midwife to develop and maintain a range of skills. These are practised and honed over a period of time unitl they become integral to her repertoire and incorporated into care seamlessly. The way that a midwife handles the newborn baby is an example of the dexterity she must demonstrate on a daily basis in order to instil confidence and gain trust from the woman and her family. Questions that arise from the scenario might include: What factors help or hinder the midwife when developing her clinical dexterity? Who acts as role model for the development of your clinical skills? How does the clinical environment influence the dexterity of your care?

Models of care

Women receive care in a range of settings depending on the options available to them and the subsequent choices that they make. Questions that arise from the scenario might include: How might this scenario have been different if Teresa had given birth in her own home? Had Teresa previously met the midwife and student who were now examining her baby? Had Teresa met the doctor who was now sitting between her legs? How does continuity of carer impact on women's experience of care? How can midwives facilitate a positive relationship and experience for women that they have not previously met?

Safe environment

Irrespective of where women receive care they need to feel that they and their baby are in safe and competent hands. They need to know that their wishes are respected and that they will be consulted before any care is instigated. Questions that arise from the scenario might include: How does the woman judge that her carers are competent professionals who are providing appropriate care? What actions might lead her to believe that she and her baby are at risk? What actions can midwives take to reassure women that they are in safe hands?

Promotes health

The postnatal period is an ideal opportunity for the midwife to promote health in both the woman and her new baby. It is a time when women are receptive to information and

advice about the best ways to care for their child and to modify their own behaviour where appropriate. Questions that arise from the scenario might include: How can midwives promote health when examining the new baby? In what ways can midwives act as role models to new parents? What healthy behaviours can women and their families adopt that will promote the health of the family? What opportunities does the doctor have to facilitate healthy behaviour during the suturing procedure?

Further scenarios

The following scenarios enable you to consider how specific situations influence the care the midwife provides. Use the jigsaw model to explore the issues raised in each scenario.

Scenario 1

Rachel is having an elective caesarean section for breech presentation. She is having a spinal anaesthetic and has written a birth plan, supported by her community midwife. In this she details how she would like to have skin-to-skin contact immediately after birth.

Practice point

Elective caesarean birth is a relatively straightforward procedure that happens in many maternity units on a daily basis. However, for the woman, it is far from routine and marks an important event – the birth of her child. Whilst it may not be possible to accommodate everyone's particular wishes, where routine care can be adapted to meet women's individual aspirations for birth, they should be considered and facilitated if possible.

Further questions specific to Scenario 1 include:

1. What do the NICE (2004) Caesarean Guidelines recommend for care of the baby born by caesarean section?
2. What are the benefits for the mother and baby of skin-to-skin contact at birth?
3. Who would need to be involved to enable Rachel to receive skin-to-skin contact with her baby?
4. Are women where you work encouraged to make a birth plan if they are having an elective caesarean section?
5. What environmental factors need to be considered when keeping a baby with its mother in theatre?
6. How can these issues be overcome?

Scenario 2

Keeley gives birth to her first baby after a long protracted labour. The baby is placed on her abdomen and she turns away and says, 'Take it away, I'm too tired.' The midwife takes the baby and dries it carefully with a warm towel, in the cot next to the bed.

Practice point

For some women the experience of birth can be a long and tiring ordeal. However, not wanting to touch or hold the baby immediately after it is born can be the

result of a combination of factors, some of which are nothing to do with how the labour and birth had progressed. The woman may prefer to have the baby cleaned up and get herself prepared to greet her new baby. She may have particular cultural practices that need to be fulfilled before she handles him.

Further questions specific to Scenario 2 include:

1. Had the midwife previously discussed with the woman how she wanted the baby to be presented to her?
2. What would you say to a woman who declines to hold her new baby?
3. How should the midwife involve the birth partner in the immediate few minutes after birth?
4. How can the midwife provide the woman with feedback about her baby if she does not want to hold him?
5. When should the midwife be concerned if the mother does not show any interest in her baby?
6. Who should the midwife inform if she has concerns about how the woman responds to her baby?

Conclusion

The immediate period following the birth requires the midwife to coordinate many important activities. S/he must facilitate successful parent–infant interaction while ensuring that key assessments and decisions are undertaken. Documentation of all observations and actions must be made to ensure safe transfer to the midwife who continues the family's care.

Resources

Baby Friendly Breastfeeding Initiative. Skin to skin contact. http://www. babyfriendly.org.uk/items/research_ detail.asp?item=98.

Birth rituals (examples). http://www. midwiferytoday.com/enews/enews0241. asp.

Cord clamping resource and information site: http://www.cordclamp.com/.

Fatherhood Institute: http://www. fatherhoodinstitute.org/.

Kangaroo care – site promoting skin-to-skin and breastfeeding. http://www. kangaroomothercare.com/.

Newborn life support. http://www. resus.org.uk/pages/nls.pdf.

Thermoregulation (Chapter). http://www.sjhc.london.on.ca/sjh/ profess/periout/chapters/ 19_thermoregulation_revised_feb_ 06.pdf.

Thermoregulation (Procedure). http://nursing.intranet.unchealthcare. org/servicelines/womens_services/ labordelivery/most-commonly-used-policies-procedures-and-protocols/ thermoregulation%20in%20the%20 newborn%20immediately%20after%20 birth.pdf.

References

Apgar V: A proposal for a new method of evaluation of the newborn infant, *Current Researches in Anaesthesia and Analgesia* 32:261–262, 1953.

Baston H, Durward H: *Examination of the newborn: a practical guide,* London, 2001, Routledge.

Carfoot S, Williamson D, Dickson R: A randomised controlled trial in the north of England examining the effects of skin-to-skin care on breast feeding, *Midwifery* 21:71–79, 2005.

Christensson K, Bhat G, Amadi B, et al: Randomised study of skin to skin versus incubator care for rewarming low-risk hypothermic neonates, *Lancet* 352(9134):1115, 1998.

DiGirolamo A, Grummer-Strawn L, Fein S: Maternity care practices: implications for breastfeeding, *Birth* 28(2):94–100, 2001.

Golding J, Greenwood R, Birmingham K, et al: Childhood cancer, intramuscular vitamin K, and pethidine given in labour, *British Medical Journal* 305(6849):341–346, 1992.

Information Centre: *NHS maternity statistics, England: 2005–2006,* The Information Centre, 2007.

McDonald SJ, Middleton P: Effect of timing of umbilical cord clamping of term infants on maternal and neonatal outcomes. DOI: 10.1002/14651858. CD004074.pub2, *Cochrane Database of Systematic Reviews* 2(CD004074), 2008.

Michaelides S: Physiology, assessment and care. In Henderson C, Macdonald S, editors: *Mayes' Midwifery. A text book for midwives*, ed 13, Edinburgh, 2004, Baillière Tindall.

Moore F: Examining infants' hips – can it do harm? *Journal of Bone and Joint Surgery* 71(1):4–5, 1989.

Moore ER, Anderson GC, Bergman N: Early skin-to-skin contact for mothers and their healthy newborn infants. DOI: 10.1002/14651858.CD003519.pub2, *Cochrane Database of Systematic Reviews* 3(CD003519), 2007.

National Institute for Health and Clinical Excellence (NICE): *Caesarean section. Clinical guideline 13*, London, 2004, NICE.

National Institute for Health and Clinical Excellence (NICE): *Routine postnatal care of women and their babies*, London, 2006, NICE.

National Institute for Health and Clinical Excellence (NICE): *Intrapartum care. Care of healthy women and their babies during childbirth. NICE clinical guideline 55*, London, 2007, NICE.

Nursing and Midwifery Council (NMC): *Midwives rules and standards*, London, 2004, NMC.

Nursing and Midwifery Council (NMC): *The Code. Standards of conduct, performance and ethics for nurses and midwives*, London, 2008, NMC.

Renfrew M, Fisher C, Arms S: *Bestfeeding: getting breastfeeding right for you: an illustrated guide*, ed 3, Berkeley, California, 2004, Celestial Arts.

Roberton N: *A manual of normal neonatal care,* London, 1996, Arnold.

Roman E, Fear N, Ansell P: Vitamin K and childhood cancer: analysis of individual patient data from six case-control studies, *British Journal of Cancer* 86(1):63–69, 2002.

Walters M, Boggs K, Ludington-Hoe S, et al: Kangaroo care at birth for full term infants: a pilot study, *MCN, American Journal of Maternal Child Nursing* 32(6):375–381, 2007.

Chapter 4

Examination of the newborn

Trigger scenario

Wendy had her bag packed and was waiting to leave the postnatal ward. Her partner arrived with the car seat and asked her if she was ready to go. She looked anxiously towards the bay entrance, 'I'm still waiting for the baby to have its examination, the midwife said I couldn't go until then.'

Introduction

All babies are offered a clinical examination within 72 hours of the birth, by a professional who has been trained to do so (Department of Health 2008). This person has traditionally been a paediatrician but increasingly midwives and neonatal nurses are undergoing additional programmes of education and supervised practice to enable them to fulfil this role (Mitchell 2003). For the purpose of this chapter,

this professional will be referred to as the practitioner. It is important that all midwives understand what the clinical examination involves so that they can discuss it with parents, both before and after the event. This chapter outlines the content of the examination and describes some of the issues that can arise from it.

What is the examination of the newborn?

As well as being checked at every postnatal examination, the newborn baby is checked systematically twice within the first 72 hours of life. The first head-to-toe examination is carried out by the midwife before she leaves the woman after a home birth or before the mother and baby are transferred from the labour ward, if birth has taken place in hospital (see Chapter 3). The purpose of that examination is to rule out gross physical abnormality

(National Screening Committee (NSC) 2008) but also provides an opportunity to reassure parents and promote health and wellbeing (Baston & Durward 2001). A subsequent examination is then performed, usually before the baby leaves hospital, ideally within 24 hours (Hall & Elliman 2006) but before the baby is 3 days old. This examination is sometimes referred to as the 'neonatal examination' (Hall 1999, Mitchell 2003), 'examination of the newborn' (Baston & Durward 2001, Townsend et al 2004), 'physical assessment of the newborn' (Lumsden 2002) or the 'newborn physical examination' (NSC 2008). Irrespective of the name given to the examination, its purpose is to detect less obvious conditions through a more detailed clinical assessment. The baby will be examined again at 6–8 weeks, as some physical conditions do not become evident until the baby is older.

and competency to undertake the role. However, in order to standardize the content of the examination performed and the competency of the individuals who undertake the examinations, the National Screening Committee (NSC 2008) has launched *Standards and Competencies* against which future commissioning should be based (Davis & Elliman 2008). The NHS for Scotland has published a Best Practice Statement (NHS Quality Improvement Scotland 2008a) which also includes core competencies and an audit form to assess compliance.

Activity

Find out how many midwives where you work conduct the examination of the newborn on a regular basis.

Ask them how many examinations they perform each year.

Who performs the examination?

There are now a range of professionals who are able to undertake the examination of the newborn – a role traditionally held by paediatricians (Lumsden 2002). Midwives and neonatal nurses must undertake further education and supervised clinical practice in order to perform this role. There are many education programmes available throughout the United Kingdom, each currently having a range of criteria for successful completion

Evaluation of the examination

When practitioners other than paediatricians started to undertake the neonatal examination, there was considerable debate as to how effective they would be, how acceptable they would be to women and what the cost implications might be (Lomax 2001). In a qualitative study exploring midwives, GPs', junior paediatricians' (Senior House Officers (SHOs)) and mothers' views (Bloomfield et al 2003), all groups felt that midwives and SHOs were appropriate professionals to carry out the examination. The majority felt that it was most appropriate for midwives to undertake the role as they had a better rapport with women and were not as rushed as SHOs. However, there was concern by some midwives about their capacity to take on additional roles within their current remit. There was little evidence of SHOs being trained for this specific examination.

In a prospective study comparing SHO referrals to specialist clinics with those from Advanced Neonatal Nurse Practitioners (ANNPs) (Lee et al 2001), it was concluded that ANNPs were more able at detecting hip and eye abnormalities. There was no difference between the professions at detecting cardiac anomalies.

In a randomized controlled trial of 826 mother and baby pairs (Wolke et al 2002), comparing paediatric SHO examination with midwife examiners, it was concluded that women were more satisfied if the examination was conducted by a midwife. This was because midwives were more likely to engage in discussion of healthcare issues. When continuity of carer and discussion of healthcare issues were taken into account, there were no differences between the groups. The study also highlighted that only 51% of newborns were eligible for examination by a midwife due to strict exclusion criteria and that midwives took about 5 more minutes than the SHO to examine the baby. In the quantitative aspect of the study (Townsend et al

2004) there were no significant differences between the doctors and midwives with regard to subsequent inpatient admissions, missing problems or referrals to consultants in the first year of the baby's life. The study also concluded that if midwives were to undertake more of the examinations, there would be a considerable saving to the NHS but some increased costs would be incurred by midwifery departments.

Activity

Consider how the midwives where you work maintain their skills in examination of the newborn.

Where and how do they provide evidence of their experience?

The examination process

It is not the remit of this chapter to prepare the reader to be able to undertake this detailed examination, but to highlight what the practitioner should include so that you can prepare the parents and understand what you observe. For a detailed explanation of the content of the examination see Baston & Durward (2001).

The neonatal examination comprises five phases (Table 4.1).

Step 1: Preparation

The practitioner should first read the case notes and assess who is the most

Table 4.1 The five steps of neonatal examination

Step	Action	Description
1	Preparation	Read case notes
		Assess who is most appropriate practitioner to undertake examination
		Explain procedure to parent(s)
		Gain verbal consent
		Listen to carers
		Gather equipment
		Wash and warm hands
2	Observation	Watch baby's behaviour
		Observe parents' behaviour
		Listen to the baby
		Listen to the parent(s)
3	Examination	Baby dressed
		Baby undressed
4	Explanation	Findings conveyed to parent(s)
5	Documentation	Examination and action documented

Source: Adapted from Baston & Durward (2001:63).

appropriate professional to undertake the procedure, in line with local guidelines. The practitioner should then approach the parents, introduce themselves and ensure that they understand what the examination entails, what they are looking for and what the procedure may not detect. Some cardiac conditions, for example, will not manifest themselves until the ductus closes (Hall 1999). Ideally, the parents should have received information during the antenatal period so that they are expecting this important screening examination. Verbal consent should be gained and the practitioner should listen carefully to any concerns that the parents may voice. The practitioner should then gather equipment (Box 4.1) and wash her hands.

Step 2: Observation

The practitioner can gain a lot of information by observing the baby's

Box 4.1 Equipment for examination of the newborn	
■ Tape measure	■ Ophthalmoscope
■ Stadiometer	■ Spatula
■ Neonatal stethoscope	■ Centile chart

behaviour and that of the parents. If awake, is the baby moving all of its limbs equally? Are there any jerky movements? What is the baby's colour? What is his respiratory pattern? Do the parents appear relaxed? Is the baby making any noise? If so, does it sound appropriate? Have the parents voiced any concerns that need to be focused on?

Step 3: Examination

Dressed

Throughout the examination the practitioner should speak to the baby and give constant feedback to the parents about her findings. She should examine the exposed parts of the baby first, to avoid disturbing him. The system requiring the most concentration is the heart, so this should be examined first over the clothes, just in case the baby cries too much when undressed later. The eyes, nose and mouth should be examined while the hands are still clean. The rooting and sucking reflex can also be elicited at this time. The head circumference and baby's length can then be measured and documented. The scalp, ears, fontanelles and shape of head are assessed next.

Activity

Identify two anomalies that might be found with the following: eyes, ears, nose, mouth, scalp, fontanelles, head.

Undressed

The baby should be gently undressed, the practitioner speaking to him all the time and observing his overall colour. Laying a warm towel or blanket over parts not to be examined, the practitioner will then go on to look at the baby's neck, hands, feet and limbs. Then the chest and heart are examined followed by gentle palpation of the abdomen. The genitalia are examined, followed by the anus, groin and hips (Fig. 4.1). The parents should be asked if the baby is feeding well and has passed urine and meconium. The baby is then turned over onto the examiner's non-dominant arm while the spine and tone of the baby are assessed. The baby's central nervous system is evaluated by an overall consideration of his behaviour, posture and tone, cry, movement and reflexes.

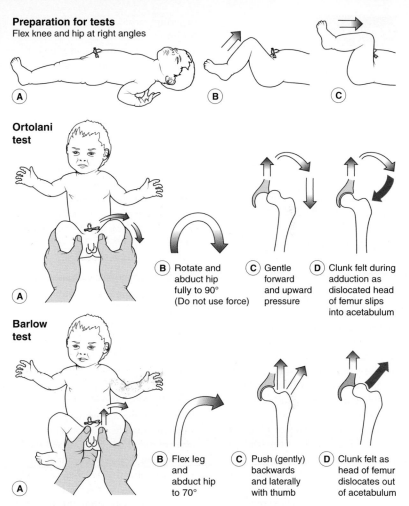

Preparation for tests
Flex knee and hip at right angles

A

B

C

Ortolani test

A

B) Rotate and abduct hip fully to 90° (Do not use force)

C) Gentle forward and upward pressure

D) Clunk felt during adduction as dislocated head of femur slips into acetabulum

Barlow test

A

B) Flex leg and abduct hip to 70°

C) Push (gently) backwards and laterally with thumb

D) Clunk felt as head of femur dislocates out of acetabulum

Fig. 4.1 Examination of the hips. (Fraser & Cooper 2003, with permission.)

Step 4: Explanation to parent(s)

It is good practice to give feedback throughout the examination but also important at the end to conclude with a final evaluation. The parents should not be left wondering; if there was any concern they should be informed in an honest and open manner, with a clear explanation of what will happen next.

Identify the two tests that are carried out on the baby's hips.

Consider what action would be taken if the baby were found to have undescended testes.

Write down the meanings of the following: the moro, stepping, palmar and plantar grasp reflexes.

Parents should always be given the opportunity to ask questions.

Step 5: Documentation

The head circumference and body length should be plotted on a centile chart, followed by documentation of the whole examination. Accurate and timely documentation of the neonatal examination is a key aspect of caring for women and their babies. It should be in a format that is accessible to all who might have a need to know the findings, including the parents, the midwives in the hospital and community, the health visitor and the general practitioner. It should detail: when, where and by whom the baby was examined, what physical characteristics and behaviours were assessed and what was found. Not all women in the UK carry their notes from hospital into the community, although there is usually a communication letter or computer printout summary of their care. The examination should be documented in the child health record. The Scottish NHS has produced a woman-held

maternity record (NHS Quality Improvement Scotland 2008b) that has a specific section for documenting all baby examinations and relevant care and maternal history.

Reflection on trigger

Look back on the trigger scenario.

Wendy had her bag packed and was waiting to leave the postnatal ward. Her partner arrived with the car seat and asked her if she was ready to go. She looked anxiously towards the bay entrance, 'I'm still waiting for the baby to have its examination, the midwife said I couldn't go until then.'

Now that you are familiar with the examination of the newborn you should have insight into how the scenario relates to the evidence about it. The jigsaw model will now be used to explore the trigger scenario in more depth.

Effective communication

Throughout the examination it is important that the practitioner is aware of their body language and the information they are transmitting by the way they stand, the faces they pull and the hesitation in their voice. Parents have a right to the information that is being gleaned and it should be fed back to them without delay. Questions that arise from the scenario might include: How long has Wendy been waiting for her baby to be examined? What information has she already been given about the examination? How has the practitioner been informed that the mother is waiting for the examination of her baby? What lines of communication are there between paediatric and midwifery staff? Have the communication systems been re-evaluated recently?

Woman-centred care

To provide woman-centred care requires the midwife to have an understanding of the woman's hopes and expectations. The midwife will also need to provide the woman with feedback about how the current maternity care systems can facilitate or sometimes frustrate the provision of individualized care. Although it may be ideal if a woman could have her baby examined in a timely manner, sometimes it is impossible because of a sudden peak in workload. If there are no midwives on duty who can perform the examination and the paediatrician has had to attend to a neonate on the Special Care Baby Unit, then the woman may need to wait. If she is provided with honest information about the situation she can modify her expectations and plans accordingly. Questions that arise from the scenario might include: Are there any midwives working in the community who might be able to undertake the examination in Wendy's home? Are there sufficient qualified practitioners to enable Wendy to choose who examines her baby?

Using best evidence

Examination of the newborn is an important screening assessment that continues to evolve as research and evaluation improves out knowledge of what constitutes effective practice. Although some aspects of the screening have a comparatively low predictive value, for example clinical examination of the hips (Zeiger & Schulz 1987), other options also have their limitations (Engesaeter et al 1990). There is no one optimum time at which all anomalies will be detected (Sherratt 2001) although undertaking the examination at 24 hours is considered optimum (Hall & Elliman 2006). Questions that arise from the scenario might include: Is there any evidence about whether waiting for examination of the newborn causes significant distress to new parents? How might this information be captured and acted on?

Professional and legal issues

It is the midwife's duty to keep up-to-date with innovations in clinical care: 'must ensure she becomes competent in any new skills required for her practice' (NMC 2004:17). Examination of the newborn is not currently requisite at the point of midwifery registration. However, if a midwife undertakes a preparation programme she is required to maintain and develop her skills in this field. Employers are also required to provide opportunities for professionals to maintain their skills if they expect their employees to use them in the course of their duties. Questions that arise from the scenario might include: How do paediatricians maintain and update their knowledge and skills in relation to examination of the newborn? Whose responsibility is it to monitor if and how midwives maintain their competence? Should professionals have protected time to keep their clinical skills up-to-date?

Team working

Providing a service that enables babies to receive the most appropriate care and intervention when needed, requires professionals to work together for that common goal. Midwives, paediatricians and neonatal nurses need to overcome any professional boundaries to ensure that they can communicate effectively about how the service can best meet their client's needs. Questions that arise from the scenario might include: What opportunities are there for midwives, doctors and nurses to learn together and share their knowledge? Are there multi-professional guidelines that enable practitioners to identify and work within their own remit and acknowledge when to refer to another? Are there clear pathways of care that facilitate effective referral?

Clinical dexterity

Achieving competence at examination of the newborn requires the midwife to gain additional clinical skills and perform them with dexterity. For example, she will need to learn to listen to the heart sounds, so that she can identify heart murmurs. She will learn how to listen to the baby's chest and identify when the respiratory system is compromised. She will need to be able

to palpate the abdomen and identify when abdominal organs appear enlarged or uncharacteristically firm. She will learn how to use an ophthalmoscope and identify the 'red reflex'. Questions that arise from the scenario might include: How will the midwife learn and master these new skills? What role models are there to help her develop effective techniques? What resources are there to enhance her learning and enable her to practise and hone her new skills?

Models of care

Enabling women to access timely and effective screening services will be influenced by the way that maternity services are configured. Models of care vary between health authorities and between hospitals and communities within the same authority. Questions that arise from the scenario might include: What provision is there for a woman to have her baby examined if she gave birth at home? Do general practitioners perform examination of the newborn where you work? Do the clinical guidelines where you work permit a midwife to examine a baby that was born by caesarean?

Safe environment

It is important that parents feel safe to disclose their worries or relevant family and/or social history during the baby's examination. It is therefore good practice to conduct the examination in a private room and/or in a manner that is sympathetic to the sensitivity raising some issues may require. Additionally, the examiner will need a well-lit, warm environment with a firm surface on which to perform the examination of the hips effectively. Questions that arise from the scenario might include: Will Wendy's baby's examination take place in the ward area or in a private room? What form of personal identification will the practitioner wear? Has Wendy received any information about not allowing a practitioner to take her baby out of her sight, unless she already knows them?

Promotes health

Examination of the newborn is an ideal opportunity to inform parents about the characteristics of a healthy baby. They can be reassured about their child's current robust health and what to look out for if they suspect that he has become unwell. It is also a time when information can be reinforced about avoiding the risk of cot death, what to look for if a baby has jaundice and whom to call if they need support. Questions that arise from the scenario might include: Will Wendy be able to make the most of the opportunity when her baby is examined or will she be distracted by the thought of her waiting partner? Will both parents be invited to be involved in the baby's examination? How can the examiner help the parents feel comfortable about asking questions and voicing their concerns?

Further scenarios

The following scenarios enable you to consider how specific situations influence the care the midwife provides. Use the jigsaw model to explore the issues raised in each scenario.

Scenario 1

Judy gave birth at home, to a healthy baby boy. It was a bank holiday weekend and her named community midwife, Claire, had gone away on holiday. Judy had hoped that her GP would be able to undertake the baby's examination.

Practice point

Not all general practitioners have maintained their skills in examination of the newborn and therefore some may be unable to undertake this assessment. Also, at the weekend, many GP practices use locum services who would not necessarily perceive neonatal examination as 'emergency' work.

Further questions specific to Scenario 1 include:

1. What contingency plans could Claire have instigated to ensure that Judy's baby had an examination within 72 hours of the birth?

2. Is it a requirement that general practitioners provide a neonatal examination service?

3. What proportion of community midwives undertake examination of the newborn where you work?

4. Do you think midwives who have not previously been involved in a woman's care should undertake the neonatal examination?

Scenario 2

Marcia has just taken up her post as a midwife in a large teaching hospital, having worked for 4 years as a neonatal examiner in a rural community team. She has been told that she cannot undertake the neonatal examination of the newborn until she has been deemed competent by the consultant paediatrician.

Practice point

From a professional point of view, if the midwife has undertaken a programme of education and supervised practice and subsequently met competency requirements, she is able to undertake the examination of the newborn. She is required to maintain her competence (NMC 2008:07) and only provide care she has been trained to undertake (NMC 2004:16). If the midwife were self-employed, she could continue to practise, providing she fulfilled her professional requirements. However, from an employment point of view, the midwife is obliged to comply with the employer's policies and guidelines. The employer may stipulate that all midwives working at that Trust who wish to undertake the neonatal examination must have their competence verified by the consultant paediatrician.

Further questions specific to Scenario 2 include:

1. Enquire about your local examination of the newborn programme. How long is the programme and how many examinations must the student undertake in order to become competent?

2. How many examinations must the midwife perform each year in order to maintain competence?

3. How should the midwife provide evidence that she has maintained and developed her clinical skills?

4. How do paediatricians maintain and develop their competence at examination of the newborn?

Conclusion

Registered midwives can undertake the examination of the newborn providing they have undergone a preparation programme and had their competency assessed. They are then required to continue to develop and maintain their skills and document their continued professional development. Midwives who perform this important screening assessment are able to enhance a woman's experience of care by providing continuity and discussing parenting and healthy living practices. Early detection of abnormality enables prompt referral to an appropriate specialist and the initiation of timely treatment.

Resources

Antenatal and Newborn screening programmes. Information leaflet for parents. http://www.screening.nhs.uk/anpublications/baby_screening_tests.pdf.

Best Practice Statement, NHS Scotland 2008. Routine examination of the newborn. http://www.nhshealthquality.org/nhsqis/files/Routine%20Examination%20of%20the%20Newborn%20BPS%202008.pdf.

Davis A, Elliman D: Newborn examination: setting standards

for consistency, *Infant* 4(4):116–120, 2008.

NHS: Newborn and infant physical examination programme. http://newbornandinfantphysicalexam.screening.nhs.uk/.

Woman's hand held record of neonatal care Scotland 2008. http://www.nhshealthquality.org/nhsqis/files/MaternityRecord_Neonatal%20Record_SWHMR_Jan2008.pdf.

References

Baston H, Durward H: *Examination of the newborn. A practical guide*, London, 2001, Routledge.

Bloomfield L, Townsend J, Rogers C: A qualitative study exploring junior paediatricians', midwives', GPs' and mothers' experiences and views of the examination of the newborn baby, *Midwifery* 19(1):36–45, 2003.

Davis A, Elliman D: Newborn examination: setting standards for consistency, *Infant* 4(4):116–120, 2008.

Department of Health: *The child health programme. Pregnancy and the first five years of life*, London, 2008, Department for Children, Schools and Families.

Engesaeter L, Wilson D, Nag D, et al: Ultrasound and congenital dislocation of the hip, *Journal of Bone and Joint Surgery* 72:197–201, 1990.

Fraser DM, Cooper MA: *Myles' Textbook for midwives*, Edinburgh, 2003, Elsevier.

Hall D: The role of the neonatal examination, *British Medical Journal* 318:619–620, 1999.

Hall D, Elliman D: *Health for all children*, ed 4, Oxford, 2006, Oxford University Press.

Lee A, Skelton R, Skene C: Routine neonatal examination: effectiveness of trainee paediatrician compared with advanced neonatal nurse practitioner, *Archives of Disease in Childhood. Fetal and Neonatal Edition* 85:F100–F104, 2001.

Lomax A: Expanding the midwife's role in examining the newborn, *British Journal of Midwifery* 9(2):100–102, 2001.

Lumsden H: Physical assessment of the newborn: a holistic approach, *British*

Journal of Midwifery 10(4):205–209, 2002.

Mitchell M: Midwives conducting the neonatal examination: part 1, *British Journal of Midwifery* 11(1):16–21, 2003.

National Screening Committee (NSC): *Newborn and infant physical examination standards and competencies.* Online. Available http://nipe.screening.nhs.uk November 3, 2008.

NHS Quality Improvement Scotland: *Routine examination of the newborn*, Edinburgh, 2008a. Online. Available http://www.nhshealthquality.org/nhsqis/files/Routine%20Examination%20of%20the%20Newborn%20BPS%202008.pdf October 30.

NHS Quality Improvement Scotland: *Scottish woman held maternity record*, 2008b. Online. Available http://www.nhshealthquality.org/nhsqis/3944.html October 31.

Nursing and Midwifery Council (NMC): *Midwives rules and standards*, London, 2004, NMC.

Nursing and Midwifery Council (NMC): *The Code. Standards of conduct, performance and ethics for nurses and midwives*, London, 2008, NMC.

Sherratt A: Working within practice boundaries: developing a parent information leaflet in order to enhance the neonatal discharge examination, *Journal of Neonatal Nursing* 7(4):120–126, 2001.

Townsend J, Wolke D, Hayes J, et al: Routine examination of the newborn: the EMREN study. Evaluation of an extention of the midwife role including a randomised controlled trial of appropriately trained midwives and paediatric senior house officers, *Health Technology Assessment* 8(14), 2004.

Wolke D, Dave S, Hayes J, et al: Routine examination of the newborn and maternal satisfaction: randomised controlled trial, *Archives of Disease in Childhood* 86:F155–F160, 2002.

Zeiger M, Schulz R: Ultrasonography of the infant hip. Part III: Clinical application, *Paediatric Radiology* 17:226–232, 1987.

Chapter 5

Hospital postnatal care

Trigger scenario

Ingrid had been having difficulty getting her day-old baby to attach properly at the breast. She had a lot of support from her midwife who helped her at each feed. The baby was awake again and rooting for a feed. As the midwife responded to her buzzer and drew the curtains around her bed, Ingrid's husband arrived with his mother.

Introduction

Hospital postnatal care is available for all women in the UK. The options given vary between maternity units and range from a few hours to several days. However, many women, especially those expecting their first baby, are often led by what the midwife recommends. Women may ask, 'What usually happens?' and the response they receive often depends on local custom and practice. This chapter describes some of the issues to consider when caring for a woman in hospital after the birth. Bathing the baby is used to illustrate the principles of teaching parents new skills through involvement and role modelling. These principles could be applied to a range of skills that new parents need to learn.

Why stay in hospital?

A hospital stay following the baby's birth may be chosen or advocated in order to address one or more of the following objectives on a 24-hour basis:

- Provide support and care to women recovering from childbirth
- Assess and monitor the wellbeing of the woman and/or her baby
- Develop and enhance parental confidence in caring for their new baby.

Each woman's needs should be individually assessed so that a package of care can be provided that meets her particular circumstances. The National

Service Framework for Children, Young People and Maternity Services (Department of Health 2004:32) requires that:

In hospital settings, each woman receives an initial assessment of her needs and agrees a care plan with the midwife which takes into account the type of birth, expected length of stay in hospital and the timing of her transfer home.

This individualized approach to postnatal care is further endorsed by the postnatal care guidelines (NICE 2006) and the government policy document *Maternity matters* (Department of Health 2007). There is evidence to suggest that midwives value providing both emotional and physical suppport to women throughout the postnatal period and see it as an important aspect of their role (Cattrell et al 2005). However, it has been reported that women are most critical of the care they receive on hospital postnatal wards than at any other time (Redshaw et al 2007). For example, only 53% of women felt treated as an individual at all times during their postnatal stay (op cit: 48).

Women's postnatal needs cannot be precisely predicted, and therefore require careful assessment following the birth. Although it is likely that a primiparous woman will take longer to feel confident handling her baby than a multiparous woman, this will not always be the case. A woman who has grown up caring for younger siblings may be very adept with all aspects of childcare, whereas one having a second baby following a long gap may take some time to regain

her confidence. The events surrounding the birth will also have an impact on whether or not the woman and her baby stay in hospital afterwards:

Mode of birth: A woman who has an instrumental birth may need time to recover from the effects of anaesthesia, a painful wound and the unanticipated intervention. In addition, a woman who has had a caesarean birth will need advice and support to recover from major abdominal surgery while mastering her maternal role (see Chapter 6).

Time of birth: A woman who had intended having a 6-hour transfer home may be advised to compromise her wishes if the baby is born in the evening.

Health of baby: A period of observation is often advocated if the baby required assistance at birth, was cold, hypoglycaemic or has a high risk of infection. Babies who become jaundiced may also require hospital care for phototherapy and careful monitoring of serum bilirubin levels. Contentiously, many NHS Trusts have policies which state that the baby's respiration rate should be closely observed (in hospital) if the liquor was meconium stained. This is particularly difficult to implement if the baby was born at home, as this would require both the mother and baby to be transferred to hospital. However, in practice, while some units have specific observation procedures, others do not and the baby remains under the observation of its mother – which, it could be argued, could be done in the comfort of their own home.

Health of woman: In a random survey of postnatal women, Glazener et al (1995) found that 85% reported at least one health problem in hospital. Many of these issues can be managed in the community setting; however, some require continued observation and treatment. For example, if a woman has had a postpartum haemorrhage (PPH) she should be closely observed for symptoms of anaemia, such as: breathlessness, syncope, lethargy and further excessive blood loss. Women with an underlying medical condition, for example diabetes or raised blood pressure, will need close observation to ensure that their drug therapy is adjusted to meet their postnatal needs.

Some women, because of current or previous psychiatric illness, will be advised to stay in hospital following the birth so that their mental health status can be closely observed. Care should be carefully coordinated and provided by the perinatal mental health team. In circumstances when psychiatric admission is required following childbirth, this should be in a specialist mother and baby unit, with her baby (Lewis 2004). Postnatal emotional wellbeing is the focus of Chapter 8.

Activity

Make sure you know the policy for estimating postnatal haemoglobin where you work.

Under what circumstances would a woman be offered iron therapy or a blood transfusion?

When it has been agreed that the woman and her baby would benefit from hospital postnatal care, her transfer to the ward should be carefully coordinated.

Transfer to the ward

Coming out of a birthing room, where the woman has some degree of privacy, onto a ward with lots of hustle and bustle, can be overwhelming. There are many ways in which the midwife can ease this transition, enabling the woman to feel part of a community rather than one of many.

Before the woman leaves the labour ward, the midwife who has been caring for her should telephone the postnatal ward to establish that there is a bed available. Brief details can be given regarding the way that the birth had progressed so that the postnatal midwife can allocate the most appropriate location. For example, some units put women who have had a caesarean delivery or who are breastfeeding together in the same bay.

If there will be a delay in transferring her, this should be explained to the woman, giving her a reason and a time by which the situation will be reviewed. When a bed is available, ideally the midwife who had looked after her should transfer her to the ward, so that a more detailed handover can be carried out. The midwife taking over her care should greet the woman by name, demonstrating that she is expecting her, and introduce herself, explaining her role and how long she will be providing her care. Baxter et al (2003) reported how some women on postnatal wards feel a sense of abandonment, often not knowing who is caring for them.

A postnatal examination of the woman should be undertaken to ensure that she is well. The baby's identity tags should be checked and its temperature taken. All observations should be documented, in the woman's presence, giving her the opportunity to ask questions and seek clarification. Any deviations from normal should be reported to the midwife who is coordinating the ward.

Introduction to the ward

Before the woman is left alone, she should receive sufficient information to enable her to summon help if she has any concerns and to know what to expect over the next few hours. The amount of detail given will depend on the time of transfer to the ward. If it is the middle of the night it may be sufficient to show her the buzzer system, where the toilet is and where and when breakfast is served. She should always feel able to buzz for assistance, whether with feeding or any aspect of baby care. It should be anticipated that she will need some help in the first few hours after the birth and while she adapts to her new surroundings. Most wards have introductory leaflets about ward routines and visiting hours that can be a useful resource for women who are unfamiliar with being in hospital.

Activity

Research the evidence on co-sleeping and bed-sharing.
 Find out the policy regarding this issue on your local maternity ward.

Single rooms

Although the thought of a single room with its own washroom facilities might sound appealing, in reality being placed alone can be quite isolating for some women. New mothers often benefit from observing how other women handle their babies; seeing that their's is not the only one that does not settle easily, or go straight to the breast without some help, can be reassuring.

However, there are circumstances when a single room away from the throng of the main ward is the best option. Women whose baby is in special care may find it difficult to be on the main ward, constantly reminded that their baby is not with them. Also, particularly if the baby is ill, she may have a constant stream of visitors who need privacy as they try to adapt to the challenge and uncertainty of the baby's condition.

Women in single rooms should be visited by a midwife regularly throughout the day. Some women do not like to ring their buzzer to ask for help when they can see how busy the staff are. Women should be encouraged to seek assistance when needed – after all, that is why they are in hospital. Ideally, women should have the choice regarding their postnatal accommodation, but availability is a limiting factor.

Security

Most maternity units have made security arrangements for the prevention of baby abduction. This may involve a combination of some or all of the following:

Locked doors: All visitors must either buzz to gain entry or have privileged access because of the nature of their work. This might be through the use of a swipe card or a keypad. Often, exit from the ward is also controlled by a similar arrangement, with visitors having to ask a member of staff to let them out.

Security cameras/videophone: A closed-circuit television camera is positioned just outside the entrance to the ward. In order to gain access to the ward, the visitor must ring a buzzer and wait for a response. The person on the ward can both see the visitor and also talk to them to establish the purpose of their visit or do the same via a telephone arrangement.

Baby tagging: There are various systems in use, and these may involve the baby having a special tag attached to its ankle that would trigger an alarm if it passed a certain point on the ward. Some wards have cots that sound an alarm when a baby is removed from it (which can be over-ridden for baby carers).

Vigilance: The most important means of protecting babies from abduction is the constant awareness of staff and parents. It is essential that you do not let anyone into the ward who cannot state a legitimate purpose for being there. For example, if a visitor says they are there to visit Mrs Jones and you are not sure if such a woman exists on the ward, then you must ask them to follow you to the desk so that you can confirm Mrs Jones' whereabouts. If they say they know where she is and promptly walk towards a bay or room, you should follow to confirm they have found the right person. If you are leaving the ward and someone is waiting outside, do not let him or her in as you exit. If you have time, ask them who they are visiting and escort them in. If not, politely ask them to ring the buzzer, stating that a member of staff will be with them shortly.

Parents and visitors should be asked to act in the same way. Although visitors sometimes have to wait for a few minutes before they are seen, they will usually welcome the safe care of the babies on the ward. Women should be informed of the professionals who might be coming to see them during their hospital stay – for example, the paediatrician or physiotherapist. They should not allow the baby to be taken away from the bedside unless they know that person. A baby should only be taken to a treatment room if a procedure is necessary that might cause the baby to cry and disturb other women, such as venepuncture. The parents should always be invited to accompany the baby.

Women should be encouraged to ask to see formal identification if they are ever unsure of someone's professional identity, and to ask a member of midwifery staff if they have any concerns. If they are going for a bath or to have a meal, they should either tell a member of staff or another mother to keep an eye on their baby.

Activity

Find out what systems are in place where you work to help prevent baby abduction.

Make sure you know the visiting times on your local postnatal ward.

Visiting hours

When a baby is born there is an intense desire to share the experience with close family and friends. Visiting time on the ward is often a flurry of pink and blue balloons and anxious parents looking for their daughter. Despite the joy and pride of showing the new baby to its admirers, there are times when the presence of visitors complicates the situation. If a woman has been having difficulties with breastfeeding, for example, she may have been on the receiving end of lots of well-meaning advice from her visitors. She may require extra support and reassurance when her visitors have left for the evening. Postnatal wards often have a time when visiting is for fathers only. Staff should respect this but there is also a need to be flexible – for example, when parents have travelled a long way

or when the baby's father is not currently part of the woman's life. Women should be encouraged to let a midwife know if there are any potential problems regarding who visits the new baby.

Recovering from vaginal childbirth in hospital

The postnatal examination

The woman and her baby should be examined daily by the midwife during her stay in hospital, but more regularly if there is any deviation from normal (see Chapter 2 for content of the postnatal examination). Women should have the opportunity to talk through the events of their labour to ensure that they understand what happened and why. In a small study (Dennett 2003) exploring women's views about having the opportunity to talk through what happened during the birth, women found it helpful to fill in the gaps and make sense of events, particularly if there were any complications. However, formal debriefing is not advocated (NICE 2006).

Length of stay

The length of hospital stay has reduced steadily over the last decade. However, there is a lack of evidence regarding the risks and benefits of early transfer home (Brown et al 2002). More than 70% of women who have a spontaneous birth leave hospital within one day of the birth (The Information Centre 2007). However women who have an instumental birth are likely to stay for 2 days. Perineal pain and discomfort is a considerable issue for women during their hospital stay.

Perineal pain

Non-steroidal anti-inflammatory drugs (NSAIDs) via suppository, given immediately after perineal suturing, are an effective analgesic for up to 24 hours after the birth (Hedayati et al 2004). However, women respond differently to analgesia and have varying degrees of laceration, oedema and bruising contributing to their individual pain or discomfort. It is important to listen to a woman who reports pain, and to find out what she has already tried to relieve her symptoms. If a woman reports severe or increasing pain, her perineum should be re-examined to ensure that a haematoma is not developing or that her wound has not become infected.

Oral analgesia followed by a warm bath is a useful means of treating mild to moderate perineal pain. The bath will help distract and then relax her while the analgesia is taking effect and also cleanse the wound. Bath additives should be avoided and a clean sanitary towel applied afterwards. A randomized controlled trial (Sleep & Grant 1988) found no difference between groups of women who were allocated to one of three 10-day bathing programmes: salt bath, Savlon bath or additive-free bathing. Cooling gel pads as a means of reducing perineal pain are highly acceptable to women (Steen & Marchant 2001) but a systematic review concluded that there is little evidence of their effectiveness (East et al 2007).

Perineal ultrasound and pulsed electromagnetic energy (PEME) are sometimes used for the treatment of a painful perineum. However, a systematic review of the limited evidence available (Hay-Smith 1998) concluded that there is insufficient evidence to evaluate the benefit or harm of such treatments, and that further research is necessary to inform practice. Similarly, there is insufficient evidence to advocate the use of topical anaesthetics for postnatal perineal pain (Hedayati et al 2005).

Activity

List any alternative therapies which are useful for the relief of perineal pain.

Find out what medications are contraindicated when the woman is breastfeeding.

Feeding the baby

For some women, the reason they have chosen to stay in hospital for a few days is so that they can become confident at breastfeeding before they go home. Women should be encouraged to ask for help if they have any difficulty latching the baby onto the breast or have sore nipples. They need to learn how to identify when the baby is latched on effectively. Just because a woman has breastfed before does not mean that she is immune to difficulties with a subsequent baby. Each child is unique and the new baby may make demands that are difficult to adjust to. When feeding is requiring a lot of support, reassurance can be given that despite the need for pillows, stools and extra pairs of hands in the first few days, breastfeeding will become second nature and soon she will be able to feed her baby and herself at the same time.

Women who have chosen to feed their baby by artificial means also require support. They will need to learn how to introduce the teat into the baby's mouth and how to hold the bottle. New mothers often worry about how much the baby is taking at each feed. Babies should be demand-fed irrespective of the method, but when fed on artificial milk should consume approximately 150–180 ml/kg/day (Roberton 1996). However, this needs translating into meaningful volumes that women can estimate. The principles of how to make up a feed and sterilize equipment should be explained on an individual basis. It is recommended that feeds are freshly made up prior to each feed rather than in batches (Food Standards Agency 2008).

Activity

Describe three methods of sterilizing bottle-feeding equipment.

Make sure you know the 10 steps of the Baby-Friendly Breastfeeding Initiative.

Gaining confidence

Looking after postnatal women requires the midwife to provide a careful mix of facilitation and care, judging when to stand back and when to step in. There is rarely a need to take over but occasionally the events surrounding birth can be overwhelming and the midwife needs to assist with all aspects of baby care.

Bathing the baby

Midwives and healthcare assistants are competent at bathing babies; they do not need any more practice. Although it is faster and simpler just to take over and demonstrate how to bath a baby, this may not be the most appropriate method of transferring skills. Some women will have experience of bathing siblings or a previous child, but may welcome reminding of the basic routine. Women also access information through friends, books and antenatal groups, and have certain ideas about how they wish to undertake this aspect of their baby's care. Preparation for childbirth classes vary in their content, and may or may not contain information about caring for the baby's hygiene needs.

The parents should be given the option of undertaking the baby's first bath, with support if required. Often, new mothers wish to observe a baby bath before they have a go themselves. Opportunities can be taken for other mothers in a bay to watch someone else's baby being bathed (with its mother's permission), but individual support – on a one-to-one basis – should also complement this experience.

The aim of doing a demonstration bath is to show the principles of caring for the baby's skin, while conveying to the woman that there are other ways of achieving the same aim. It is not about her being able to replicate, move by move, the technique that you demonstrate, but her finding a way that is comfortable for her. Where possible, the baby's father should be invited to take part in this social event.

Principles of bathing a baby

Special time together: Bathtime for babies often becomes part of a bedtime routine that involves close contact between the baby and its parents. With this aim in mind, efforts should be made to ensure that bathtime is associated with warmth, closeness and lots of attention. All parents have busy lives, but bathtime is an opportunity to share games and cuddles, and can be an oasis in an otherwise frenetic day. From the first bath onwards, the baby should be talked to and given personal attention and eye contact to help make the experience pleasurable.

Timing: When babies are very young, and routines are not established (or desired), bathtime is probably more likely to be based on a need to clean the baby than anything else. Babies do not need a bath every day, but it is a great opportunity to make sure that s/he is not getting sore anywhere. Sometimes

it may be the easiest way to clean a baby, following a particularly soiled or leaked nappy, for example. Finding the best time of day can be difficult to get right. It is not advisable to bath a baby who has just been fed, as this may lead to regurgitation and bowel movement (necessitating another bath!). Bathing a baby who is very hungry is likely to be distressing for all concerned. Choosing a time when the baby is alert and content, and also when there are unlikely to be interruptions, would be the ideal situation.

Keeping the baby warm: Newborn babies have an immature thermoregulation system (Michaelides 2004). They are particularly vulnerable to heat loss via evaporation when wet, hence the place where babies are bathed should be draught-free and warmer than usual. Delay during the bathing process can lead to the baby cooling down, so it is important that all equipment is to hand before the baby is undressed (see Box 5.1 for equipment checklist).

A range of equipment is used in hospital, from a formal baby bath on a stand to a washing-up bowl that can be placed on a table. Only about 8 cm of water is required: more than this would be heavy and difficult to carry. The bath water should be 37°C, and is commonly tested by dipping the elbow into the water (which should feel warm – not hot or cool).

Removing matter from the face and neck: The baby should be undressed down to its nappy and wrapped in the towel. One way of doing this is to turn a corner of the towel down and, with

---

Box 5.1 Baby bath equipment checklist

- Warm, dry towel
- Change of clothes
- Clean nappy
- Cotton wool
- Barrier cream
- Baby shampoo/bath additive/soap
- Baby bath or equivalent
- Changing mat

---

this newly created edge at the nape of the baby's neck, swaddle the baby by wrapping one point of the towel round its body and under its back and the other point around the other side.

The first part of the bath is cleansing the baby's face. This should be done using cotton wool, dipped in the bath water (additives are not recommended, NICE 2006) and squeezed to remove excess water. One side of the face is done at a time to avoid the possibility of conferring infection from one side to the other. A firm but gentle action starts at the middle of the forehead, moving around the eye (but never across it), round to the nose, back across the cheek, around the ear, then around the mouth. A second piece of dry cotton wool follows the same track. The same process is repeated for the other side of the face. Then another piece of damp cotton wool should be used to clean under the baby's neck. It will be necessary to use one hand to gently extend the baby's chin upward to reveal the baby's neck. This area should then be carefully dried.

Removing debris from the hair: The baby's hair should be washed next, and with a small baby this is easiest if the baby is held under the non-dominant arm, its head supported by the hand. This leaves the dominant hand free to do the washing. A bath additive can be introduced to the water at this point. The baby is then held over the bath and the dominant hand used to cup water and release over the head. The hair and scalp should be gently rubbed using the pads of the fingers to loosen any debris, and fresh water from the bath used to rinse it away. It is important not to take too long washing the hair and to dry it promptly. This can be done by turning up the corner of the towel at the nape of the neck and rubbing the head firmly.

Inspecting skin folds: The baby's nappy should now be removed and cotton wool used to remove any soiling from the buttocks.

Now the baby is ready to go into the bath: With the baby on the lap with its head resting across the non-dominant arm, the baby's distal arm should be

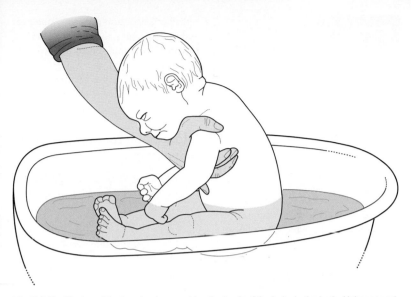

Fig. 5.1 Positioning of the hands when washing the back of the baby in the bath. (Johnson and Taylor 2006, with permission.)

grasped using the non-dominant hand. Then the baby's distal leg should be grasped using the dominant hand with the forearm supporting the proximal leg. It sounds complicated, but using this method the person holding the baby has a firm grasp and can place the baby into the water. Keeping the non-dominant hand in the same position supporting the baby's head, the dominant hand can be used to wash the baby. When it is time to wash the baby's back, the baby can be sat up and the grasp on the distal arm transferred to the other hand so that the baby can be leant over the dominant forearm while the non-dominant hand is used to do the washing (Fig. 5.1).

When the bath is finished, the baby should be dried quickly, paying particular attention to skin folds. A thin coating of barrier cream can be applied around the anus. If disposable nappies are being used, further application to the buttocks should be avoided as this can prevent the absorption of urine. The baby should then be dressed, and equipment cleared away and cleaned.

Examination of the newborn

Before the baby is transferred to the community, a thorough clinical examination is undertaken, usually within the first 24–72 hours. The purpose is to reassure parents that their baby is healthy and has no abnormalities (Baston & Durward 2001). This examination is performed either by a midwife or nurse who has undertaken a programme of further education and practice to gain competence with this skill, or by a paediatrician. Where possible, the baby should be examined with the parents present so that they can ask questions and be involved in the process. Observing this examination, with the parents' permission, is an excellent opportunity for the student midwife to learn about neonatal behaviour and health. See Chapter 4 for further details of this important screening examination.

Newborn hearing screening test

Between one and two babies in every thousand are born with a hearing loss of some kind (Newborn Hearing Screening Programme (NHSP) 2008). All babies are offered hearing screening, usually before they leave hospital, but sometimes in GPs' surgeries, community clinics or in the baby's home. It involves the insertion of a soft

tipped ear piece into the baby's outer ear and monitoring of the baby's response to sound, by a trained hearing screener. The results are given to the parents immediately afterwards and many babies require a further screening test due to inconclusive results.

Information for parent before going home

Many hospital Trusts have a checklist of issues the midwife should discuss with the woman prior to transfer into the community. These include:

- Advice regarding safe sleeping practices (see Chapter 7 for details)
- Contraceptive advice (see Chapter 9 for details)
- Registering the birth (see Chapter 7 for details)
- When to contact a doctor
- Community midwifery contact details
- Safe transport of the baby
- Giving the woman her postnatal notes
- Explaining any continuing drug therapy
- Postnatal support helplines.

Leaving hospital

Taking the new baby home is a time of mixed emotions for many new parents. It is a time of great excitement but also a time when parents acknowledge the responsibilities they face for the next 18 years. The aim is that they leave hospital feeling confident in their abilities, yet aware of the support that they can obtain if required.

Reflection on trigger

Look back on the trigger scenario.

Ingrid had been having difficulty getting her day-old baby to attach properly at the breast. She had a lot of support from her midwife who helped her at each feed. The baby was awake again and rooting for a feed. As the midwife responded to her buzzer and drew the curtains around her bed, Ingrid's husband arrived with his mother.

Now that you are familiar with hospital postnatal care you should have insight into how the scenario relates to the evidence about it. The jigsaw model will now be used to explore the trigger scenario in more depth.

Effective communication

There is so much information to convey to a new mother and it is important that she understands what the midwife is saying and the rationale behind her advice. Every effort should be made to ensure that communication between the midwife and woman is effective and that information is reinforced in a variety of ways. Questions that arise from the scenario might include: How much information did Ingrid receive about postnatal care and routines in hospital? When did she receive it and in what format? Did Ingrid share the information with her partner? How did the midwife respond to the arrival of visitors at this time?

Woman-centred care

This involves a sensitive, individualized approach to care and consideration of the woman's needs over and above those of her carers. Providing woman-centred care might also mean that the midwife needs to take account of the woman's family and their role in her adaptation to motherhood. Questions that arise from the scenario might include: How can the midwife ensure that Ingrid receives the care and support she needs without alienating her family? What information does the midwife need in order to involve other members of the family in an appropriate manner? What actions could the midwife have taken to avoid any awkward situations at visiting time?

Using best evidence

To provide effective care to women the midwife must use her knowledge regarding the most appropriate means and method for supporting women to breastfeed in the context of the woman's individual circumstances. Where possible, care should be based on the best available evidence (NMC 2008). Questions that arise from the scenario might include: Did the midwife provide a rationale for the advice that she was giving Ingrid? Is there any evidence to suggest that length of hospital postnatal stay has any influence on the duration of breastfeeding? What is the evidence to support baby-led feeding? What are the sources of evidence for woman and midwives regarding the initiation and continuation of breastfeeding?

Professional and legal issues

Midwives must practise within a professional and legal framework to maintain high standards of care and protect women from potential harm. The professional standards of conduct outlined in The Code (NMC 2008) also require midwives to act as advocates for those in their care. To evaluate the scenario further you might consider the following issues: How much information should midwives disclose to a woman's relatives? In which professional guidance does it indicate that it is the midwife's role to support women feeding their baby? Did the midwife ask Ingrid's consent prior to drawing the curtains around her bed? Did the midwife document the care she gave Ingrid?

Team working

Though midwives are often the sole providers of postnatal care in hospital, they are members of a wider team with skills to support women from a range of perspectives. It is important that they communicate with each other: each may have a particular insight into a woman's situation. Questions that need to be addressed in this scenario are: Is the midwife always the most appropriate person to provide support to breastfeeding women? Are there any indications that Ingrid and her baby need to be referred to another professional or peer supporter? If so, who might this be? Where will the midwife record information for other members of the team to access and contribute to? How will the midwife make contact with other health professionals if required?

Clinical dexterity

In this scenario the midwife will require skill and experience to support Ingrid to feed her baby. The midwife will need to recognize when the baby has successfully latched on to Ingrid's breast and how well the baby is feeding. Questions that could arise: Has the midwife received appropriate training in the skills required? What opportunities are there for qualified midwives to update their skills for supporting women to breastfeed? How will the midwife help Ingrid maintain her privacy and dignity throughout the feed? How will she maintain her skills and pass them on to others?

Models of care

Midwives provide postnatal care in a range of settings. How care is organized is likely to influence the way that care is provided. Receiving hospital-based postnatal care may not always be the most family friendly model of care; however, it may also have some advantages. Questions that arise from the scenario might include: Is Ingrid close to home or have her relatives travelled a long way, coping with public transport or congested car parks, in order to visit? How would Ingrid have accessed support with breastfeeding if she had had a home birth? Who is available to support the midwife who is providing care? What resources are available in the hospital that are not available in the community, to support women to breastfeed?

Safe environment

Midwives work in a variety of locations and need to assess the risks each environment may present. Ensuring that the woman and her baby do not come to any harm during their postnatal stay in hospital is paramount. Supporting women to breastfeed can present unanticipated challenges to the safety of the environment. For example, if the woman needs to undress in any way in order to provide an unrestricted access to her breasts, she is at risk of losing dignity. If she is feeding her baby in bed, she risks falling asleep with potentially fatal consequences. Questions that arise from the scenario might include: What steps can the midwife take to maintain Ingrid's dignity throughout the care she provides? How can she ensure that she is positioned correctly for optimum comfort of the woman and herself? Did the midwife wash her hands in between clients? What measures can the midwife take to reduce the risk of Ingrid falling asleep whilst feeding her baby?

Promotes health

Hospital postnatal care provides many opportunities to promote the health and wellbeing of both the woman and her family. Whilst it is a time that women are keen to seek information and ask for advice, it is also a time when the provision of so much information can be confusing and overwhelming. Questions that arise from the scenario might include: Did the midwife explain the benefits of breastfeeding for Ingrid and her baby's health, both now and

in the future? Does Ingrid know how to access other sources of support for feeding her baby? Has Ingrid been shown how to recognize when her baby is feeding well at the breast and what other indicators will give her confidence that her baby is receiving adequate nutrition? Does Ingrid understand when it would be important to seek the help of a health professional?

Further scenarios

The following scenarios enable you to consider how specific situations influence the care the midwife provides. Use the jigsaw model to explore the issues raised in the scenario.

Scenario 1

Marianne has had an instrumental birth following delay in the second stage of labour. The following day her perineum has become very painful. She tentatively tries to get out of bed but finds that moving her legs is too painful. She winces with pain. The woman in the next bed goes to her and says, 'You need a salt bath, I swear they helped me after my first.'

Practice point

Perineal pain can be debilitating and frightening for some women. There are many helpful remedies, from the use of warm water to oral analgesia, so it is important that the woman feels that she can ask for support and intervention if necessary. A certain degree of pain is expected when there is a perineal wound. Feeling this pain may be delayed as the woman may have had an epidural or local analgesia at the the time she incurred the trauma. She is also likely to have had a suppository containing a NSAID at the time of the perineal repair and when this wears off, the wound can feel heavy and swollen and throb with pain. It is important that the midwife excludes the development of haematoma or infection if women complain of severe perineal pain during the postnatal period.

Further questions specific to Scenario 1 include:

1. Why is salt in bath water no longer recommended for the treatment of perineal pain?
2. What would be your first line of management if you were caring for Marianne?
3. How long would you expect a perineal wound to take to heal?
4. Why is it important to provide effective analgesia for women who have perineal pain?
5. What alternative remedies have been shown to be effective in reducing perineal pain and bruising?

Scenario 2

Gabi was transferred from the labour ward to the postnatal ward in a wheelchair, holding her baby tightly. Jane, a healthcare assistant, took her to the midwives station. A midwife looked up and said, 'Hello, you must be Gabi Jones. I am Hannah and I will be looking after you tonight. Jane, would you settle Gabi into bay 6 and I'll be right with you.'

Practice point

Leaving the close observation of the labour ward can be rather daunting. The relief that was felt following the safe arrival of the baby can be overshadowed for a while by an uncertainty about what will happen next. This is an important time of transition as the new parents get to know their baby and they face the realization that they now have to provide everything for this dependent infant. Knowing that they will be cared for by someone who will take time to get to know them and their individual needs can make this time one of joyful discovery. Alternatively, if their arrival on the ward is met with lack of knowledge or interest, the night ahead can seem interminable.

Further questions specific to Scenario 2 include:

1. How is information about women and babies to be transferred from the labour ward to the postnatal ward, conveyed where you work?
2. Does this system work well or can you identify how it could be improved?
3. Where does the handover of care take place?
4. What are the advantages and disadvantages of this activity taking place at the woman's bedside?
5. Do women where you work have a choice regarding single room or bay accommodation: which option would you choose and why?
6. What is the role of maternity support workers in hospital postnatal care at the Trust where you work?

Conclusion

The midwife working on the postnatal ward must assess when to observe and support women caring for their babies and when to step in and teach by example. The needs of postnatal women alter as their confidence grows and they recover from the birth. The aim is that she leaves the ward feeling well and happy and looking forward to the first night at home with the baby.

Resources

Breastfeeding helplines. http://www.breastfeeding.nhs.uk/en/fe/page.asp?n1=4.

Guidance for health professionals on safe preparation, storage and handling of powdered infant formula. http://www.food.gov.uk/multimedia/pdfs/formulaguidance.pdf.

Healthy Start, advice for professionals. http://www.healthystart.nhs.uk/en/fe/page.asp?n1=1&n2=8.

Making up a bottle feed. Advice sheets in different languages. http://

www.babyfriendly.org.uk/page.asp?page=115&category=5.

Newborn hearing screening. Questions and answers for professionals. http://www.hearing.screening.nhs.uk/cms.php?folder=206.

Sterilizing feeding equipment. Advice sheets in different languages. http://www.babyfriendly.org.uk/page.asp?page=115&category=4.

References

Baston H, Durward H: *Examination of the newborn. A practical guide*, London, 2001, Routledge.

Baxter J, McCrae A, Dorey-Irani A: Talking with women after birth, *British Journal of Midwifery* 11(5):304–309, 2003.

Brown S, Small R, Faber B, et al: Early postnatal discharge from hospital for healthy mothers and term infants DOI: 10.1002/14651858.CD002958, *Cochrane Database of Systematic Reviews* 3(CD002958), 2002.

Cattrell R, Lavender T, Wallymahmed M, et al: Postnatal care: what matters to midwives, *British Journal of Midwifery* 13(4):206–213, 2005.

Dennett S: Talking about the birth with a midwife, *British Journal of Midwifery* 11(1):24–27, 2003.

Department of Health: *National Service Framework for children, young people and maternity services. Standard 11*, London, 2004, Maternity Services.

Department of Health: *Maternity matters: choice, access and continuity of care in a safe service*, London, 2007, Department of Health.

East CE, Begg L, Henshall NE, et al: Local cooling for relieving pain from perineal trauma sustained during childbirth DOI: 10.1002/14651858. CD006304.pub2, *Cochrane Database of Systematic Reviews* 4(CD006304), 2007.

Food Standards Agency: *Guidance for health professionals on safe preparation, storage and handling of powdered infant formula*, 2008. Online. Available http://www.food.gov.uk/multimedia/pdfs/formulaguidance.pdf October 19.

Glazener CM, Abdalla M, Stroud P, et al: Postnatal maternal morbidity: extent, causes, prevention and treatment, *British Journal of Obstetrics and Gynaecology* 102(4):282–287, 1995.

Hay-Smith E: Therapeutic ultrasound for postpartum perineal pain and dyspareunia DOI: 10.1002/1465185. CD000495, *Cochrane Database of Systematic Reviews* 3(CD000495), 1998.

Hedayati H, Parsons J, Crowther C: *Rectal analgesia for pain from perineal trauma following childbirth (Cochrane Review)*, The Cochrane Library, Chichester, 2004, John Wiley.

Hedayati H, Parsons J, Crowther CA: Topically applied anaesthetics for treating perineal pain after childbirth DOI: 10.1002/14651858.CD004223. pub2, *Cochrane Database of Systematic Reviews* 2(CD004223), 2005.

Information Centre: *NHS Maternity Statistics, England: 2005–2006*, The Information Centre, 2007.

Johnson R, Taylor W: *Skills for midwifery practice*, ed 2, Edinburgh, 2006, Elsevier.

Lewis GE: *Confidential enquiry into maternal and child health. Improving the health of mothers, babies and children. Why mothers die 2000–2002. Midwifery summary and key recommendations*, London, 2004, RCOG.

Michaelides S: Physiology, assessment and care. In Henderson C, Macdonald S, editors: *Mayes' Midwifery. A text book for midwives*, ed 13, Edinburgh, 2004, Baillière Tindall.

National Institute for Health and Clinical Excellence (NICE): *Routine postnatal care of women and their babies*, London, 2006, NICE.

Newborn Hearing Screening Programme: *About newborn hearing screening*, 2008. Online. Available http://www.hearing.screening.nhs.uk/ October 31.

Nursing and Midwifery Council (NMC): *The Code. Standards of conduct, performance and ethics for nurse and midwives*, London, 2008, NMC.

Redshaw M, Rowe R, Hockley C, et al: *Recorded delivery: a national survey of women's experience of maternity care*, Oxford, 2007, National Perinatal Epidemiology Unit.

Roberton N: *A manual of normal neonatal care*, London, 1996, Arnold.

Sleep J, Grant A: Effects of salt and Savlon bath concentrate post-partum (not full paper), *Nursing Times* 84(21):55–57, 1988.

Steen M, Marchant P: Alleviating **perineal** trauma – the APT study, *RCM Midwives Journal* 4(8):256–259, 2001.

Chapter 6

Postoperative care following a caesarean

Trigger scenario

Jasmine's baby was crying. Her legs were still wobbly following a spinal anaesthetic administered for her emergency caesarean. She looked around her trying to remember what the midwife had said about calling for assistance if she needed it. The midwife had told her how lucky she was to have a room to herself.

Introduction

The caesarean birth rate in the United Kingdom is currently 23.5% (The Information Centre 2007) – more than a fifth of all births. The challenge for midwives caring for a woman following caesarean section is to acknowledge that she has undergone not only the birth of her baby but also major surgery, both of which are significant life events. Supportive care that enables the woman to recover from her surgery while mothering her new baby requires the midwife to judge astutely when to stand back and observe and when to step in and offer assistance. Such care must be adapted to meet the needs of individual women, each having their own hopes and fears of both parenthood and recovery from surgery. This chapter describes both hospital and community postnatal care following caesarean birth, and outlines care additional to that described in Chapter 5, 'Hospital postnatal care'.

Immediate postnatal care

Prophylactic antibiotics

Before the woman leaves theatre she will have received a prophylactic dose of antibiotics. As the Confidential Enquiry into Maternal and Child Health (CEMACH) report *Saving Mothers' Lives* (Lewis 2007) states, puerperal infection is the second highest cause of maternal death, and the risk is increased following emergency caesarean section. Hofmeyr & Smaill (2002) undertook a systematic review to assess the effectiveness of antibiotic therapy in reducing the incidence of infection following caesarean delivery due to a reduction of endometritis by between two-thirds and three-quarters; they concluded that all women undergoing caesarean section should receive antibiotic therapy.

Hopkins and Smaill (1999) explored which drug regime is most appropriate: they found that ampicillin and cephalosporins had similar efficacy, and that one dose in theatre was probably sufficient. They recommended that further research be undertaken in order to clarify whether it should be given before or after the cord is clamped.

Postoperative recovery

When the woman comes out of theatre there is a period of close observation or 'recovery' during which regular observations of respiration, heart rate and blood pressure are made. Initially these are recorded every 5 minutes, but as the woman's condition resumes normal parameters they will become less frequent (every 15 minutes, then half-hourly). In addition to the above observations, the woman's temperature and level of pain are noted. Her wound will be observed for bleeding and her pad examined for assessment of lochia. An intravenous infusion will be in progress and her urinary catheter observed for the expected diuresis following childbirth. All observations should be meticulously documented

and any deviation from normal reported to a senior midwife.

The woman should have one-to-one care until she can maintain her own airway, can communicate and is cardio-respiratorily stable (Association of Anaesthetists 2002, NICE 2004). Following transfer to the ward area (often labour ward initially) her observations should be recorded every half hour for 2 hours then hourly if satisfactory. It is particularly important to monitor the woman's respiration rate if opioids have been administered (NICE 2004).

General anaesthesia

If the woman was asleep for the birth of her baby, she will require close observation as she recovers from the anaesthetic. It is important to be aware that she will be able to hear what is going on around her before she is able to talk to you. It is important, therefore, that messages about the wellbeing of the baby are conveyed to her before she opens her eyes. If her birthing partner is with her, then he should be encouraged to tell her the news about the baby. She will recognize his/her voice and this will be reassuring for her.

Following general anaesthetic the woman may be drowsy but her level of consciousness should gradually improve. She may feel nauseous, in which case the anaesthetist should be informed and anti-emetics prescribed and administered. Her level of pain should be continually assessed, and supplementary analgesia given as necessary. She should not leave the recovery area until she can maintain her own airway, is fully conscious and has nausea and pain under control (Association of Anaesthetists 2002).

Epidural/spinal anaesthesia

Following surgery under regional anaesthetic, the woman should feel comfortable and alert. She may be very tired, however, if the birth was preceded by a long labour, and may wish to rest rather than plunge into her mothering role. Until the effect of the anaesthetic wears off she will have reduced sensation in the lower half of her body and will thus not automatically be able to adjust her posture to alleviate the discomfort of pressure from the hard recovery trolley. She should therefore be assisted to change position regularly and her pressure points should be observed for evidence of redness (reactive hyperaemia).

Activity

Identify the reasons why women have a general anaesthetic for their caesarean birth.

Consider how you would respond to a woman who informed you that she was afraid of being awake during surgery.

Analgesia

Assessing pain levels is an integral part of postoperative care. The woman should be encouraged to inform a midwife as soon as any pain begins to return. This should be clearly distinguished from

'let us know if you need any tablets', because once this situation has been reached the woman will have expended unnecessary energy on coping with pain rather than enjoying her baby. Effective analgesia is also important to aid a safe postoperative recovery. When a woman is in pain she is less likely to be fully mobile. She may curl up around her scar and not feel comfortable enough to undertake leg and deep breathing exercises. She will be reluctant to walk to the toilet and her general level of mobility will be reduced, increasing her risk of venous thrombosis. When a woman is experiencing wound pain she may lack confidence to handle her baby and find breastfeeding too much to contemplate.

A non-steroidal anti-inflammatory drug (NSAID) given rectally in theatre has been shown to be an effective means of reducing the use of opioids postoperatively (Lim et al 2001). Subsequent pain managed with a combination of oral NSAIDs and paracetamol, rather than just oral paracetamol, has been shown to reduce the use of morphine administered via patient-controlled analgesia in the first 24 hours after caesarean (Munishankar et al 2008).

Activity

Read the recommendations in the NICE guidelines (2004) regarding analgesia following caesarean delivery.

List the contraindications for non-steroidal anti-inflammatory drugs (NSAIDs).

Continuing care

Support to mother

If the woman had a general anaesthetic, she should be reunited with her baby and partner as soon as possible. If she had a regional anaesthetic, they should not have been separated, unless the baby required resuscitation. She will need assistance to undertake her role as mother, and every effort should be made to help her achieve this in accordance with her wishes. For example, before the baby was born she may have had ideas about what she wanted the baby to be dressed in to meet its first visitors. Where appropriate, the woman should continue to make the decisions she would have made if the baby had been born vaginally. She should know how to summon help and be encouraged to do so.

Feeding the baby

Women who wish to breastfeed should be helped to do so as soon as practicable after the baby's birth. This may mean asking the mother if she wishes to feed her baby while she is in the recovery area. This can be achieved in a lying position and will require the constant presence of a knowledgeable carer. The mother will still have an intravenous infusion in her arm at this point and will need help dealing with her theatre gown and holding her baby. The opportunity to feed the baby while she is most alert should not be missed (irrespective of method of feeding) and will give her confidence to enjoy future feeds. However, if the mother is unable to feed during this time, she should be reassured that breastfeeding will still be established.

As already mentioned, it is essential that the woman is pain free so that she can focus her attention on enjoying the feed. NSAIDs are not contraindicated during breastfeeding and during the time when opioids are more likely to be used by the mother, lactation is not established. Thus, it has been suggested that there is little evidence to support the restricted use of opioids at this time (Hestenes et al 2008).

Mobility and prophylaxis against thromboembolism

Depending on when the baby was born and on her general condition, the woman should be encouraged to get out of bed within a few hours. When sitting in a chair, the legs should be positioned on a stool to avoid additional strain on the abdominal muscles. When walking, care should be taken to ensure that the back is straight and that the woman is looking ahead, not down.

Venous thrombosis and thromboembolism (VTE) remain the highest cause of direct maternal death (Lewis 2007). The audit reported 15 postnatal direct deaths attributed to VTE, 7 of which were after caesarean section. Although abdominal surgery presents its own risk, it is the accumulation and coincidence of other risk factors that necessitate caution when caring for women who have caesarean deliveries. For example, the woman may have had a long labour and enforced immobility due to epidural analgesia prior to the birth. In the early postnatal period, she will be less mobile than a woman who has had a vaginal birth. Other factors, such as obesity, infection, multiparity and age over 35 years, also increase the risk of VTE.

Each woman should be assessed for her individual risk of VTE and offered prophylactic treatment accordingly. The Royal College of Obstetricians and Gynaecologists (RCOG 1995) recommends that women who have had elective surgery and are otherwise well with no other risk factors (i.e. low risk) should be encouraged to mobilize early and ensure adequate hydration. Women who have had emergency caesarean or who have another risk factor, such as obesity, are deemed 'moderate risk' and should be offered one form of prophylaxis. Women who have three or more risk factors or who have had a complicated caesarean experience are 'high risk' and should receive both heparin prophylaxis and possibly leg stockings.

A systematic review (Gates et al 2002) concluded that there was insufficient evidence regarding the best method of thromboprophylaxis after birth. Using decision analysis, Quinones and colleagues (2005) concluded that pneumatic compression stocking reduced the risk of VTE without increasing the risk associated with heparin prophylaxis and was the most appropriate method to use.

Fluid balance and dietary intake

The woman can drink sips of water within an hour of her baby's birth and eat as soon as she feels hungry, provided there are no complications (NICE 2004). In a systematic review comparing early oral fluids versus delayed fluids (Mangesi & Hofmeyr 2002) the authors concluded that caesarean may not disrupt bowel function and there is no evidence to recommend withholding food or drink after caesarean. The woman's intravenous infusion can be discontinued the day after the birth provided that her urinary output has been adequate and oral fluids have been well tolerated. The urinary catheter can also be removed the next day or as soon as the woman is mobile, at least 12 hours after her last epidural top-up (NICE 2004).

Personal hygiene

When the woman has had a chance to spend some time with her new family she may appreciate help with a refreshing wash before she is inundated with visitors. A change of clothes, face wash, brush of teeth and perineal toilet will suffice initially. On the next and subsequent days it will be easier for the woman to shower rather than bathe following surgery, as she may find it difficult to get in and out of the bath. Assistance should always be offered as she may also find it difficult to stand, walk and carry her wash things while holding her abdominal wound.

Wound care

The dressing should be removed from the wound the day after the birth and inspected to ensure that it is dry and the skin edges are in close proximity. The woman should be encouraged to look at it, as her expectations may be much worse than reality. She should be reassured that the skin will usually be healed within the week, although it will take longer for the underlying tissues to recover.

It is probably appropriate at this point to ask the woman what she understands about the process involved in order to deliver her baby abdominally. An explanation can help her understand the sensations she experienced during the birth and help dispel misconceptions.

Activity

Consider what factors influence wound healing.

Describe the phases of wound healing.

Define the terms 'primary and secondary intention' in relation to wound healing.

Length of hospital stay

Length of stay following caesarean section has been reported to be between two and four days, irrespective of whether surgical birth was planned (The Information Centre 2007). However, the caesarean section clinical guideline (NICE 2004) states that women who are apyrexial, are recovering and have not had any complications can be offered early discharge (after 24 hours).

Ideally, a woman should be able to decide when she feels ready to go home. This will depend on her confidence regarding the care of her baby in conjunction with her physical capacity to undertake this role. The latter will be mediated by the support she has at home. Going home on day two is probably less feasible for a woman who has had a long labour, a general anaesthetic and a toddler to contend with than for a primigravida following elective surgery under spinal anaesthetic. However, individual women will have their own hopes, concerns and support systems. Some women enjoy being in hospital, feel reassured by the 24-hour availability of support and make lifelong friends during their stay. Other women yearn for the comfort and privacy of their own home and aim to return as soon as physically possible.

Special care babies

For some mothers, recovery from surgery is compounded by the need to visit a sick or premature baby in a special care environment. The woman had probably not anticipated needing an emergency caesarean and it may have been undertaken with little time to adjust to the idea. If the baby then required specialist care, she may be left feeling shocked and bewildered.

Keeping information flowing is essential. The woman will need to be given an honest assessment of her baby's condition and to be involved in decisions about his or her care as appropriate. A member of special care staff should visit her as soon as possible with an update on the baby's progress and with a photograph that she can keep with her. These early photographs become an integral part of the memories and birth story that is remembered and retold over the years. When it is not possible for her to visit the special care baby unit herself, the midwife can make enquiries on the woman's behalf or, with the use of portable phones, enable the woman to communicate directly with the nurse or midwife who is caring for her baby. As soon as the woman can sit in a wheelchair she should be taken to see her baby and encouraged to touch and talk to him/her. Simple explanations of the monitoring equipment and treatment her baby has received should be provided. She might wish to keep a diary of key events to help her remember her baby's early days since life in hospital can become timeless as each day rolls into the next. Photographs will aid this process and should be encouraged.

Activity

Consider how you would explain to a woman, in simple terms, the process of delivering her baby by caesarean section.

Talking about the birth

The woman should be clear about the reasons why she had a caesarean section and have the opportunity to discuss any gaps in her recall of events. She should have the opportunity to discuss the reasons for the caesarean before she goes home (NICE 2004). The delivery records will facilitate this, and adequate time should be given to this aspect of postnatal care. The woman should be encouraged to ask for clarification about her surgery. One study (Dennett 2003) suggested that women valued talking about the birth later once more pressing concerns about the baby had been resolved.

Talking about the birth should be distinguished from the intervention 'debriefing' which has not been shown to reduce the incidence of postnatal depression 6 months after the birth in women who had an operative birth, and may even contribute to psychological morbidity (Small et al 2000).

Caring for the baby at home

There are aspects of baby care that require careful thought following abdominal surgery, especially when bending is involved. Bathing the baby, for example, can be particularly difficult, and should ideally be done when someone else is around. The woman should not attempt to carry a bath full of water and should avoid bending over a bath at a low level. Not only are the abdominal muscles recovering from being separated during surgery but the ligaments in the woman's back are also softened because of the influence of progesterone during pregnancy. This means that she is susceptible to injury following heavy lifting.

Placing the bath on a sturdy, protected table and standing while bathing the baby is one way of avoiding low-level bending. Also, nappy-changing facilities can be organized at a comfortable height for the first few weeks. All equipment should be gathered close to hand before the baby is placed on a high piece of furniture to avoid the temptation of leaving the baby unattended in order to retrieve a forgotten item.

Removal of stitches

Surgeons vary in the way they choose to close the abdominal wound. Some prefer a continuous, sub-cuticular stitch; others, interrupted stitches or clips. They can be removed as soon as the wound is healed, hence individual assessment is required prior to removal. The wound is usually healed within five days but may take longer in some women. If the wound starts to gape following removal of a suture, no further sutures should be removed. It may be necessary to refer the woman back to her obstetrician if there is no sign of healing.

The technique for removing sutures is a clean one and is based on the principle that no suture that has been outside the skin should be taken inside. So the stitch should be lifted by the knot, using the non-dominant hand, and cut close to the skin (using disposable scissors or a blade) with the dominant hand. Clips require special clip-removers, the lower blade of which is inserted under the clip and the handle squeezed together in order to straighten the clip and release it from its grasp on the skin edges (see Fig. 6.1).

Driving

Women have traditionally been told that they should not drive for at least 6 weeks after a caesarean birth. The rationale for this advice was that using the foot pedals involves the abdominal muscles and there should be no impediment to this aspect of driving, especially in terms of being able to make an emergency stop. NICE guidance (2004) states that women can resume driving when pain is no longer an impediment.

Housework

Even in a household where domestic chores are shared equally, the weeks following caesarean delivery are a time when the woman should be exempt from certain tasks. In the first couple of weeks, vacuuming and hanging out the washing should be avoided. Other chores such as carrying heavy baskets of washing and loading the car with shopping should be avoided for at least 6 weeks (until the effect of progesterone on the ligaments has diminished).

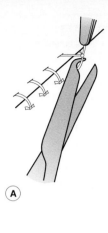

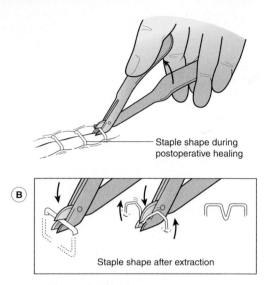

Staple shape during postoperative healing

Staple shape after extraction

Fig. 6.1 A Removing sutures. (Adapted from Jamieson et al 2002.) **B** Removing staples. (Adapted from Lammon et al 1995.)

Postnatal exercises

Postnatal exercises are particularly important after a caesarean delivery, as they will also help prevent complications following surgery. Each maternity unit will have its own schedule of postnatal exercises, often designed and administered by obstetric physiotherapists. In the first few days following the birth, exercises should include deep breathing, leg exercises and pelvic floor exercises.

Deep breathing

This exercise serves a dual purpose. Following general anaesthetic there is the potential for secretions to build up in the lungs. This is exacerbated if the woman is in pain and taking shallow breaths. Following adequate analgesia and supporting her abdomen with a cushion, she should be encouraged to take a few slow, deep breaths every hour. This will not only help clear her lungs but also aids venous blood to return to the heart, thus aiding circulation.

Leg exercises

It is important that venous blood circulation is maintained in order to prevent thrombosis. Circulation can be improved by undertaking regular leg exercises, such as rapid ankle rotations, pointing and pulling up the toes and pressing and releasing the backs of the knees into the bed (Fletcher 1991).

Activity

What is the mechanism by which deep breathing and leg exercises aid venous return?

List five non-physical benefits of taking regular exercise.

The woman should be informed of the rationale behind any advice she is given. Although it may be alarming to be told that she has an increased risk of VTE, she has the right to be aware of this so that she can make an informed choice about whether or not to undertake the exercises.

Pelvic floor exercises

Pelvic floor exercises are encouraged for the prevention and treatment of stress incontinence. Although less of a problem for women who have had one or two caesarean sections (Wilson et al 1996), risk factors such as obesity, older age and multiparity can contribute to the prevalance of this problem (MacArthur et al 1993). These exercises should be undertaken throughout life and practised regularly in groups of about six, aiming for at least 50 a day (Fletcher 1991). A systematic review of the effectiveness of pelvic floor exercise (Hay-Smith et al 2008) concluded that they are an appropriate treatment for women with postnatal urinary incontinence.

Possible long-term sequelae of caesarean delivery

Most women who have a caesarean birth do not suffer long-term problems. However, women who have emergency caesarean sections are reported to have a higher incidence of postnatal depression (Boyce & Todd 1992), low self-esteem (Marut & Mercer 1981, Fisher et al 1997) and have low emotional wellbeing postnatally (Green et al 1998). Subsequent pregnancy is less likely following a caesarean delivery (Garel et al 1990, Murphy et al 2002), and there is an increased risk of placenta praevia if conception is achieved (Hemminki & Jouni 1996).

Bainbridge (2002) states that women often come away from a previous caesarean section with the need to 'get it right' next time. However, some women opt for elective caesarean section, determined not to go down the same route of medicalized labour ending in surgery (Ryding et al 1997).

Reflection on trigger

Look back on the trigger scenario.

Jasmine's baby was crying. Her legs were still wobbly following a spinal anaesthetic administered for her emergency caesarean. She looked around her trying to remember what the midwife had said about calling for assistance if she needed it. The midwife had told her how lucky she was to have a room to herself.

Now that you are familiar with care of the baby at birth you should have insight into how the scenario relates to the evidence about this aspect of the midwife's role. The jigsaw model will now be used to explore the trigger scenario in more depth.

Effective communication

For the woman to feel safe after her caesarean section, she needs to know that she can summon help if she needs it. Providing a single room for a woman may give her privacy and an opportunity to rest. However, for some women, being alone can be frightening and isolating. Questions that arise from the scenario might include: What was Jasmine told before she was left alone, caring for her new baby? If you were in hospital, how easy would you find it to pull the buzzer? What factors might make it easier to ring for help? What factors might prevent Jasmine asking for help?

Woman-centred care

For a woman to receive individualized care, based on her perception of need, her unique situation should be assessed by the midwife who cares for her. Taking time to identify how she feels and what her expectations are can enhance her postnatal hospital experience. Questions that arise from the scenario might include: Had Jasmine been in hospital before? How might that experience influence how she feels now? Does Jasmine know how to settle her crying baby? How have Jasmine's individual needs been assessed and accommodated?

Using best evidence

It is important that maternity services evolve in the light of the best available evidence, to prevent care becoming ritualistic and routine. If there is robust evidence that one particular practice is better than another, we need to audit that aspect of care and evaluate whether that care is actually being given. Questions that arise from the scenario might include: Is there any research that explores the most appropriate place for women to be cared for in the first few days after caesarean birth? Does the phenomenon 'demanding patient' exist in maternity services? Is there any research evaluating the impact of women sharing a room with their partner whilst in hospital?

Professional and legal issues

Jasmine's midwife has a duty of care to both Jasmine and her baby. She must always act in their best interests and ensure that the care she provides is in line with current best practice. The midwife should ensure that she seeks consent before all procedures and treats Jasmine with respect. Questions that arise from the scenario might include: Was Jasmine asked if she wanted to be cared for in a single room? What provision did the midwife make to ensure that Jasmine could access professional help if required? If a student midwife was also caring for Jasmine, who would be professionally accountable for her care?

Team working

Many different professionals and support workers contribute to the care of a woman following caesarean birth. Some of this work will be carefully coordinated whereas some might be haphazard and opportunistic. The different members of the healthcare team should know what their contribution is, how it can best be executed and when referral to another carer will be the most appropriate action for the woman. Questions that arise from the scenario might include: Who is most likely to answer the buzzer if Jasmine rings for help? How often will Jasmine's named midwife 'pop in' to see how Jasmine is feeling? Would someone enter the room only if they had a specific task to do?

Clinical dexterity

Caring for a woman following caesarean birth requires considerable clinical dexterity. There are a number of clinical interventions that might be required during the course of her postnatal recovery. Jasmine will have had her clinical observations taken many times since she came out of theatre; she will need her epidural cannula, her intravenous infusion line and urinary catheter removing, all of which require the employment of the appropriate procedure and technique. Questions that arise from the scenario might include: How do midwives learn to perform skills with confidence and compassion? Are midwives dexterous when they can undertake a skill without

thinking or when they perform skills with thought?

Models of care

All women who have a caesarean birth will experience hospital postnatal care, but how that care is delivered will depend on the local model of care. In some maternity units, care is allocated bay by bay, others work in teams dependent on the consultant or the geographical location. When the woman leaves hospital, care may be given in the woman's own home, GP surgery or local children's centre. Questions that arise from the scenario might include: How is postnatal care organized where you work? How might Jasmine benefit from a team approach to care? What are the advantages and disadvantages for midwives who work in teams?

Safe environment

The provision of a safe and effective service is the goal of all maternity provision. However, this should not mean that care is provided in a ritualistic manner. Principles of safe care can be adapted to meet the individual requirements of women. Environments can be adapted to enable women to continue to provide care, for example, when they cannot bend or stand for long periods. Questions that arise from the scenario might include: What provision has the ward made to ensure that Jasmine's baby is cared for in an environment that is safe and secure? How is the risk of cross infection (between women, babies, staff and relatives) reduced on the postnatal ward where you work?

Promotes health

To regain and maintain postnatal health, women need access to information about the activities that will have a positive impact on their recovery. For example, women need to be shown how to do leg exercises to promote venous return, but they also need to understand why this is important. A woman may choose not to do an exercise because she does not understand the point in it; she might not take the same stance if she knew it could prevent her from developing a deep vein thrombosis. Questions that arise from the scenario might include: What information had Jasmine been given to enable her to make healthy choices about her postnatal recovery? Who else could be involved in Jasmine's recovery process? What is the optimum timing for a subsequent pregnancy?

Further scenarios

The following scenarios enable you to consider how specific situations influence the care the midwife provides. Use the jigsaw model to explore the issues raised in the scenario.

Scenario 1

Ruth gave birth to a baby girl by caesarean section, five days ago. She had noticed that her wound had begun to gape

at one end and was leaking fluid. She was finding it quite painful to hold her baby to feed, as she rested on her abdomen.

Practice point

Wound infection is a potential complication of all abdominal surgery and requires prompt recognition and treatment. Infection is related to the number of vaginal examinations in labour, emergency procedures, length of operation and previous history of wound infection (Webster 2008).

Further questions specific to Scenario 1 include:

1. How is a wound infection diagnosed?
2. How is a caesarean wound infection treated?
3. What are the consequences of having a wound infection?
4. What lifestyle factors are related to an increased risk of wound infection?
5. What is a stitch abscess?
6. What advice can the midwife give women to reduce the risk of developing a wound infection after caesarean birth?
7. Do wound drains help prevent infection after caesarean birth?

Scenario 2

Hazel was feeling great, two days after her emergency caesarean section. She held her baby close, amazed at how perfect she was. She looked up as her sister entered the room. After a brief greeting and mutual adoration of the new arrival, her sister said, 'You look so happy. I really thought you would be so disappointed having to have a caesarean after all those natural childbirth classes you went to.'

Practice point

Whilst women are less likely to give a positive appraisal of their birth experience if they have a caesarean, the majority of women are satisfied and do not suffer any negative long-term consequences. One of the most important factors contributing to a positive birth experience is the attitude of caregivers and the interactions and relationships they have with women in their care.

Further questions specific to Scenario 2 include:

1. How do antenatal expectations relate to postnatal experiences?
2. Can you identify three ways that the midwife can help the woman feel positive about her caesarean birth?

3. What opportunities are there for women where you work, to have a say in the management of their birth experience?
4. Are birth partners 'allowed' in theatre where you work, if their partner is having a general anaesthetic for her caesarean?
5. Do you think women should be able to observe the birth of their baby by caesarean? Why?

Conclusion

Caesarean birth presents a considerable challenge for the woman endeavouring to care for her new baby. Midwives have the opportunity to help her fulfil her role through gentle support and understanding. A quiet, unobtrusive presence combined with vigilant observation skills are required to help her achieve a fulfilling start to her new family life.

Resources

Association of Anaesthetists of Great Britain and Ireland: Perioperative management of the morbidly obese patient. http://www.aagbi.org/publications/guidelines/docs/Obesity07.pdf.

Breastfeeding within one hour of birth (Gupta 2007). http://www.ibfanasia.org/Article/Initiating_breastfeeding_within_one_hour.pdf.

Gates S, Anderson ER: Wound drainage for caesarean section. DOI: 10.1002/14651858.CD004549.pub2,

Cochrane Database of Systematic Reviews 1(CD004549), 2005.

Intra-operative cell salvage. http://www.nice.org.uk/nicemedia/pdf/ip/IPG144guidance.pdf.

Royal College of Obstetricians & Gynaecologists: Thromboembolic disease in pregnancy and the puerperium: acute management, 2007. http://www.rcog.org.uk/resources/Public/pdf/green_top_28_thromboembolic_minorrevision.pdf.

References

Association of Anaesthetists: *Immediate postanaesthetic recovery*, London, 2002, The Association of Anaesthetists of Great Britain and Ireland.

Bainbridge J: Choices after caesarean, *Birth* 29(3):203–206, 2002.

Boyce P, Todd A: Increased risk of postnatal depression after emergency caesarean section, *Medical Journal of Australia* 157(3):172–174, 1992.

Dennett S: Talking about the birth with a midwife, *British Journal of Midwifery* 11(1):24–27, 2003.

Fisher J, Astbury J, Smith A: Adverse psychological impact of operative obstetric interventions: a prospective longitudinal study, *Australian and New Zealand Journal of Psychiatry* 31(5): 728–738, 1997.

Fletcher G: *The National Childbirth Trust. Get into shape after childbirth*, London, 1991, Ebury Press.

Garel M, Lelong N, Marchand A, et al: Psychosocial consequences of caesarean childbirth: a four-year follow-up study, *Early Human Development* 21(2): 105–114, 1990.

Gates S, Brocklehurst P, Davis LJ: Prophylaxis for venous thromboembolic disease in pregnancy and the early postnatal period. DOI: 10.1002/14651858.CD001689, *Cochrane Database of Systematic Reviews* 2(CD001689), 2002.

Green J, Coupland V, Kitzinger J: *Great expectations. A prospective study of women's expectations and experiences of childbirth*, Hale, 1998, Books for Midwives Press.

Hay-Smith J, Mørkved S, Fairbrother KA, et al: Pelvic floor muscle training for prevention and treatment of urinary and faecal incontinence in antenatal and postnatal women. DOI: 10.1002/14651858.CD007471, *Cochrane Database of Systematic Reviews* 4(CD007471), 2008.

Hemminki E, Jouni M: Long-term effects of cesarean sections: ectopic pregnancies and placental problems, *American Journal of Obstetrics and Gynecology* 174(5):1569–1579, 1996.

Hestenes S, Hoymork S, Loland B, et al: Do women with caesarean section have to choose between pain relief and breastfeeding? (Abstract), *Tidsskr Nor Laegeforen* 128(19):2190–2192, 2008.

Hofmeyr GJ, Smaill FM: Antibiotic prophylaxis for cesarean section. DOI: 10.1002/14651858.CD000933, *Cochrane Database of Systematic Reviews* 3(CD000933), 2002.

Hopkins L, Smaill F: Antibiotic prophylaxis regimens and drugs for cesarean section 1002/14651858, *Cochrane Database of Systematic Reviews* 1(10), 1999.

Information Centre: *NHS Maternity Statistics, England: 2005–2006*, The Information Centre, 2007.

Jamieson EM, McCall JM, Whyte AW: *Clinical Nursing Practice*, ed 4, Edinburgh, 2002, Churchill Livingstone.

Lammon CB, Foote AW, Leli PG, et al: *Clinical nursing skills*, Philadelphia, 1995, WB Saunders.

Lewis GE: *The confidential enquiry into maternal and child health (CEMACH). Saving mothers' lives: reviewing maternal deaths to make motherhood safer – 2003–2005. The seventh report on confidential enquiries into maternal deaths in the United Kingdom*, London, 2007, CEMACH.

Lim N, Lo W, Chong J, et al: Single dose diclofenac suppository reduces post-cesarean PCEA requirements, *Canadian Journal of Anesthesia* 48: 383–386, 2001.

MacArthur C, Lewis M, Bick D: Stress incontinence after childbirth, *British Journal of Midwifery* 1(5):207–215, 1993.

Mangesi L, Hofmeyr GJ: Early compared with delayed oral fluids and food after caesarean section. DOI: 10.1002/14651858.CD003516, *Cochrane Database of Systematic Reviews* 3(CD003516), 2002.

Marut J, Mercer R: The cesarean birth experience: implications for nursing, *Birth Defects, original article series* 17(6):129–152, 1981.

Munishankar B, Fettes P, Moore C, et al: Combination of diclofenac and paracetamol, *International Journal of Obstetric Anesthesia* 17:9–14, 2008.

Murphy DJ, Stirrat G, Heron J, et al: The relationship between caesarean section and subfertility in a population-based sample of 14541 pregnancies, *Human Reproduction* 17(7):1914–1917, 2002.

National Institute for Health and Clinical Excellence (NICE): *Caesarean section. Clinical Guideline 13*, London, 2004, NICE.

Quinones J, James D, Stamilio D, et al: Thromboprophylaxis after cesarean delivery. A decision analysis, *Obstetrics and Gynecology* 106(4): 733–741, 2005.

RCOG: *Report of a Working Party on prophylaxis against thromboembolism in gynaecology and obstetrics*, London, 1995, RCOG.

Ryding EL, Wijma B, Wijma K: Posttraumatic stress reactions after emergency cesarean section, *Acta Obstetrica et Gynecologica Scandinavica* 76(9):856–861, 1997.

Small R, Lumley J, Donohue L, et al: Randomised controlled trial of midwife led debriefing to reduce maternal depression after operative childbirth, *British Medical Journal* 321(7268):1043–1047, 2000.

Webster J: Post-caesarean wound infection: a review of the risk factors, *Australian and New Zealand Journal of Obstetrics and Gynaecology* 28(3): 201–207, 2008.

Wilson P, Herbison R, Herbison G: Obstetric practice and the prevalence of urinary incontinence three months after delivery, *British Journal of Obstetrics and Gynaecology* 103:154–161, 1996.

Chapter 7

Postnatal care in the community

Trigger scenario

Vanessa had been in hospital for two days following the birth of her first child by ventouse extraction. She returned home to a sink full of dirty dishes, over-flowing bins and an empty fridge. Her partner went out again to return the car he had borrowed from his mate. She slumped onto the sofa holding her sleeping daughter and closed her eyes.

Introduction

Adjusting to life at home with a new baby can be overwhelming (Hunter 2004). This chapter outlines some of the issues faced by new parents as they care for their babies at home, and considers how the midwife can ease this transition. It describes some of the information needs of parents and the issues that midwives need to consider during their postnatal visits. The example of 'weighing the baby'

is used to illustrate how the midwife needs to make an individual assessment of the woman and her baby, before she undertakes what might be considered routine care.

National Service Framework

The National Service Framework (NSF) for Children, Young People and Maternity Services (Department of Health 2004), Standard 11 'Maternity Services', outlined radical changes to maternity care. Traditionally, midwives had visited women following their baby's birth for between 10 and 28 days (United Kingdom Central Council (UKCC) 1998). However, following changes to the Midwives Rules (NMC 2004:07), the postnatal period is now 'not less than 10 days and for such longer period as the midwife considers necessary.' The NSF (Department of Health

2004:33) reinforced this change by recommending that:

…midwifery-led services should provide for the mother and her baby for at least a month after birth or discharge from hospital, and up to three months or longer depending on individual need.

The NSF also recommended that if extra care is required for a woman, a maternity support worker could provide it. Under the supervision of either a midwife or health visitor, and having received appropriate training, this person can be part of the 'community postnatal care team' and be able to provide general advice on issues including feeding and hygiene. A study undertaken by King's College (2007) concluded that maternity support workers have varied roles and have the potential to make a positive contribution to women's care.

Activity

Find out about the support offered to postnatal women in the Netherlands.
    Find out how the 'Sure Start' initiative has contributed to women's postnatal wellbeing.

Transfer home

The length of postnatal hospital stay in the UK varies depending on the mode of birth. Women who have unassisted vaginal births stay in hospital an average of one day, those having an instrumental delivery one to two days, and those who

have a caesarean two to four days (The Information Centre 2007). This short stay means it is essential that the woman receives sufficient information to enable her to feel confident caring for her baby. Although she and her baby are being discharged from hospital, her care is being transferred from one midwife to another – hence, 'transfer to community care' is a more accurate description of this event.

Before the woman leaves hospital it is important that she is reminded about some vital public health issues. These points should also be reinforced by the community midwife following the woman's transfer home.

Baby's sleeping arrangements

Sudden infant death syndrome (SIDS) or 'cot death' accounts for the death of 340 babies each year in the UK (Foundation for the Study of Infant Deaths (FSID) 2006a). There are many steps that parents can take to minimize the risk. Box 7.1 summarizes the main points highlighted in the leaflet for parents, *Reduce the Risk of Cot Death* (Department of Health 2007).

Back to sleep

This means that babies are put to sleep on their back, not on their front or on their side. The midwife needs to alert the woman that friends and relatives of an older generation who are also involved in the baby's care may previously have been advised to put babies on their side and supported in this position with a rolled-up blanket

> **Box 7.1** Minimizing the risk of sudden infant death
>
> - Baby should be placed on its back to sleep
> - Baby should be put to bed in the 'feet to foot' position
> - Do not overheat: the baby's head should be uncovered indoors and the bedroom temperature set at 18°C
> - Provide a smoke-free environment
> - Baby to sleep in cot in parents' room for first 6 months
> - No bed-sharing if parents are over-tired, have been drinking alcohol, taking drugs or are smokers
> - Settle to sleep with a dummy
> - Seek prompt medical advice if baby appears unwell

or towel against their back. The woman should be advised, therefore, to pass on these recommendations to all those who will be involved in caring for the baby.

The principle behind placing the baby on its back to sleep is that this is the best position to allow the baby to lose heat, due to the larger surface area of the abdomen. When babies are on their front or wedged on their side with a blanket they cannot lose as much heat and can become too warm. Although it is important to keep babies warm, especially the newborn, a temperature of 18°C in the bedroom is adequate, covering the baby with two light blankets. It is therefore useful if parents have a thermometer they can use to show the true temperature of the baby's environment rather than leaving this aspect of care to chance.

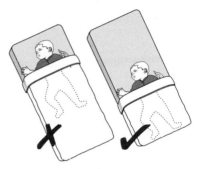

Fig. 7.1 'Feet to foot' sleeping position. (From Fraser & Cooper 2003, with permission.)

over its covers prevents him or her slipping down below them (Fig. 7.1). Although it looks strange, and not like the traditional image of the new baby in its cot, this measure could prevent the baby from dying due to suffocation or overheating.

'Feet to foot'

Placing the baby to sleep with its feet at the foot of the cot before pulling

Smoke-free zone

Babies who live with parents who smoke are 30% more likely to have a cot death than babies who live in a smoke-free environment (FSID 2006b). Although it may be distressing for parents who smoke to be told this, they have the right to this information and the opportunity to alter their behaviour and that of others. If they choose to continue to smoke they should be advised not to do so in the same room as the baby and to ask visitors to leave the room if they wish to smoke.

Settle to sleep with a dummy

There is evidence to suggest that babies who go to sleep sucking on a dummy have a reduced incidence of cot death (McGarvey et al 2003). However, breastfeeding babies should not be offered a dummy until 1 month of age, to enable feeding to be well established before a teat is introduced.

No sleeping on sofa

When a baby is unsettled during the night, there is a temptation for some parents to take the baby downstairs so as not to disturb other family members. Feeding the baby on the sofa when a parent is tired is a very risky practice as there is a strong possibility that they will both fall asleep. So that the baby does not roll off the sofa, parents are likely to put the baby between themselves and the sofa back, and if the baby slips down there is a risk of suffocation. It would probably be more prudent for the parent who is trying to sleep to find an alternative bed for the night (on the sofa) than the parent whose turn it is to feed or settle the baby.

Seek medical advice

If the baby appears unwell, it is appropriate that parents are encouraged to seek medical advice, irrespective of the time of day. New parents are often concerned that they will not recognize when their baby is ill, and a few general tips can be suggested to them. The midwife can use the baby to demonstrate characteristics of good health. If the woman recognizes a healthy baby, she will soon detect when her baby is unwell.

Is the baby well?

Colour: New babies are often pale but their lips and nail beds should be pink. Some babies develop jaundice (yellow discoloration of the skin) when they are a few days old. If this happens when the baby is less than 24 hours old, parents should seek immediate medical advice. Most jaundice is physiological and provided the baby is alert and demands regular feed does not usually require treatment. The midwife will monitor babies with jaundice but parents should seek advice in between visits if the baby becomes reluctant to feed, if its skin or sclera (whites of the eyes) become more yellow or if it passes pale stools (NICE 2006).

Tone: Well babies have a flexed tone and move all limbs equally.

Behaviour: A baby that is well will demand regular feeds. It should not have a high-pitched cry, tremble or twitch. It should pass urine at least every 5 hours (Hilton & Messenger 1991) and only have loose, frequent stools if breastfeeding. Advice should be sought if the baby starts to vomit.

Temperature: The baby should be warm to the touch, but not hot or cool – the tummy is a good place to test (Department of Health 2007). Well babies do not sweat. If the woman is concerned that her baby is either too hot or too cold she can take its temperature using a thermometer suitable for use on babies (not a mercury and glass one). The normal temperature for babies is between 36.5°C and 37.2°C (Baston & Durward 2001), and advice should be sought if there is any concern, particularly if there are other signs of ill health.

Intuition: Sometimes it is difficult to put a finger on what is wrong with a baby, but if parents have any concerns they should seek advice either from the maternity service (if still under their care) or general practitioner. Out-of-hours calls are sometimes referred to NHS Direct for advice.

Activity

Make sure you understand what causes physiological jaundice.
    Find out when and how jaundice is treated.

The first night at home

The first night at home with a new baby is an exciting new journey. The awareness that parents are alone in the house with a baby who is totally dependent on them for every need can be a stark realization and result in worry and concern. Questions will run through their minds, such as, how long will the baby sleep, will I be able to settle her/him after a feed, what if I don't hear the baby cry? It can also be a time of utter joy, and the adoration of the new family member can take up many wakeful hours.

Midwife's first postnatal visit

The midwife is informed by the hospital of the woman's transfer home, and writes her name, address and birth details in her diary for a visit the following day. It is rare for the midwife to be asked to go the same day, but this may happen if, for example, the woman has gone home early with a small baby before feeding has been established or if there has been some concern that needs monitoring.

Midwives who work in the community also run antenatal clinics and undertake other duties such as parent education classes and booking interviews. Hence, midwives visits are undertaken around other commitments and the woman needs a general idea of when to expect a postnatal visit. If a long delay is anticipated, the community midwife can use her mobile phone to keep the woman informed.

After home birth

Depending on when the baby was born, the midwife will visit again to assess progress. For example, if the baby was born in the morning it might be appropriate to visit again later in the afternoon to see if the baby is demanding milk and passing urine and meconium. If the woman had her baby in the evening, she should be seen the next morning.

Student midwives in the community

For a student on the first community placement, visiting women in their own homes can be an awkward time. Not only are you having to form a relationship with your mentor, spending time together driving around the area trying to ask intelligent questions, but you are also fighting the humiliation of feeling stupid and ignorant. But fear not. Most midwives can remember vividly how they felt when they were starting out, and understand what it feels like to sit on the sofa next to a mentor, not knowing if or when to speak.

Midwifery mentors do not expect you to know the latest research on breastfeeding or how to recognize postnatal depression, but they do expect you to be polite and communicative with the woman. How good you are at this when you begin your midwifery programme will depend on your personality and previous experience. But it is a skill that you will need to develop quickly if you do not already have it. It is quite usual to feel awkward but a friendly smile and a 'Hello, my name is Becky' is a simple way to start. You can agree with your mentor in the

car how to handle introductions. For example, the midwife introduces herself and then you say who you are and that you are working with her for the next few weeks.

As the placement progresses you will be visiting women whom you have already met at antenatal clinic. This element of continuity will quickly make you realize how important this is in community care. You will remember each individual woman's concerns – for example, that she was worried she was carrying a huge baby and anxious about the birth. It will be interesting for you to see how labour worked out for her and how big the baby actually was (you will probably have palpated her abdomen and made an assessment yourself).

What you actually do during the visit will depend, to some extent, on the stage you are at within your midwifery programme and the learning outcomes you need to achieve. However, it will also depend on how enthusiastic you are to learn and how interested you appear. Mentors vary and you may need to be quite explicit about your learning needs. For example, if you have seen your mentor take out stitches before, you can ask her about the procedure in the car. You can then ask if she will talk you through it next time or watch you while you do it, depending on how confident you feel. The rule is that you should never do something that you have not been shown how to do, no matter who asks you. This applies to qualified midwives too (except in an emergency) (NMC 2004:16).

Activity

Find out how information about the woman and her baby is communicated from the hospital to the community where you work.

The morning after the night before

When the midwife and student (if applicable) arrive at the woman's home, they introduce themselves to the family. Community midwives usually provide postnatal care for women on their own caseloads, but occasionally they visit women whom they have not previously met whose own midwives are on days off, on holiday, sick or caring for a woman in labour.

Women vary in terms of how they adjust to the additional family member. Some take it in their stride and are up and dressed the next day as if it were any other – with the baby washed, fed and dressed and sleeping soundly when the midwife arrives. In the first week the above scenario is rare. Many households take time to catch up with their new arrival and are likely to be surrounded by a plethora of equipment, visitors and evidence of the previous evening's meal. It is quite common for the woman to spend most of her time caring for the baby and not getting round to her own shower until lunchtime.

It is important that the midwives do not pass judgment on the tidiness or otherwise of the woman's home. We only have a glimpse into people's lives and do not always know the full picture regarding the pressures that many women live with. However, where there is a situation that could potentially be hazardous to the health of either the woman or her baby then the midwife must address it. For example, if the room is full of smoke, parents must be strongly advised to keep areas where the baby is cared for a 'smoke-free zone'. Or where there are animals in the house, the parents need to be reminded to make sure that the cat does not snuggle down in the baby's pram. An experienced midwife does not look around the house reeling off a list of 'don't do this and don't do that' but, especially if the woman is one of her caseloads, will quickly build up a rapport that enables her to judge how to say what.

The postnatal examination

The woman will leave the hospital with documents that provide the community midwife with relevant information about the birth and subsequent recovery. This takes many different forms, ranging from the actual birth records to a hand-completed transfer form. Many maternity units use computerized transfer letters, and the details are then transferred to a postnatal care document.

Activity

What is the Edinburgh postnatal depression scale?
Find out about the various groups in your area for women with new babies.

The elements of the postnatal examinations for both the woman and her baby are outlined in Chapter 2. The first visit at home after the birth is an important one for the community midwife as she will make observations that form the basis of her subsequent care. She is likely to undertake most of the possible elements of a postnatal examination to assure herself that she has made a thorough assessment of the woman's current health status and that no potential cause for concern has been missed.

The same is true in terms of examining the baby. It may be that a condition has developed between the previous examination in the hospital and the first one at home: for example, the baby may have become jaundiced. Depending on local policy, the baby may come home with a supply of vitamin K for oral administration. The midwife should ensure that the woman is aware of the regime and how to give the vitamin to the baby. All observations are documented in the records, which will remain with the woman.

This first visit from the community midwife is also important for the woman. She may have lots of questions, and she should be encouraged to write them down for subsequent visits so that she does not forget issues that she needs information about. She should be given the opportunity to recount her birth story and to ask questions about events that occurred during labour that remain unclear. It is important that misconceptions are clarified as this story will be retold many times over the years, with the potential to impact on future generations.

If the woman is breastfeeding it is valuable if the community midwife can observe a feed, particularly if the woman is experiencing sore nipples or engorgement. Positioning and attachment at the breast is crucial to ensure that the baby feeds effectively and without causing pain and damage to the mother. The midwife can show the woman and her partner how to recognize when the baby is feeding well and what to do if not. If the woman reports problems with feeding, it may be necessary to return to her later in the day to find out if the suggestions have helped or if further advice is required. Hanss (2004:387) writes about her experiences as a new breastfeeding mother and how she needed support in person rather than on the end of a phone:

Telephone support can be useful for basic advice, but it is impossible to assess breastfeeding technique or the health of the baby over the telephone.

Activity

Explain why vitamin K is offered to all babies.

Find out about the regime for vitamin K administration where you work.

Research the evidence to support the administration of vitamin K to all babies.

Pattern of visiting

There is no set number of visits although many Trusts will have guidelines that midwives can use as a framework. Ideally, the midwife will continue to visit according to the needs of the woman and following discussion with her. It is more likely that women who have had a baby before will require fewer visits, but this should never be assumed. A midwife who carries a caseload of women is in the fortunate position of being able to get to know the woman before she has her baby. She therefore has the opportunity to develop a relationship with her, which means that the woman feels comfortable asking for help if needed and the midwife feels confident that this will indeed be the case. The woman is given a contact number, usually the maternity unit, which she can phone if she has any 'in-between visit' problems.

Subsequent visits

Assessment of wellbeing

Following the birth, there are so many issues for the woman to deal with that some problems do not come to the surface until others have resolved. Some problems can be masked by remedies for others. For example, if a woman has been taking regular analgesia for perineal pain, once that has resolved and she stops taking her painkillers she may become uncomfortable with backache. The midwife should continue to encourage postnatal exercises and provide information about local groups where mothers can take their new babies.

The midwife should continue to provide the opportunity for a woman to raise issues of concern regarding her health. Emotional support is particularly valued, especially when time is taken to find out exactly how a woman is feeling (Singh & Newburn 2001). The issue of postnatal emotional wellbeing is addressed in Chapter 8.

Activity

Consider the reasons why babies lose weight in the first few days after birth.
Make sure you know when they should regain their birthweight.

Weighing the baby

Parents and grandparents are often concerned about the baby's weight, and see this as an important indicator of health. However, as midwifery practice becomes more evidence based, babies are being weighed less often. It is now thought – particularly if the baby is being breastfed – that attention to weight may cause more anxiety and lead women to worry that their baby is not getting enough milk. Of, course, the opposite can also be the case. A woman who has been struggling with feeding can be reassured by seeing her baby's weight increase and can also use this information to reassure sceptical relatives that she is supplying her or him with sufficient sustenance. Thus, the decision regarding the best time to weigh a baby can be a complex one to make.

Most babies lose weight in the few days after birth (Wright & Parkinson 2004). This is normal unless weight loss is more than 10% of the birthweight (Roberton 1996). After this time the baby should gain approximately 30 g per day (Roberton 1996) and have regained its birth weight by day 10 (Johnson & Taylor 2006). As with so many aspects of maternity care, not all maternity units advocate the same practice. Even where there is an evidence-based guideline in place, individual midwives exercise their professional discretion in its interpretation. This makes life confusing for the student midwife who is attempting to learn 'best practice'. However, experience enables the midwife to anticipate and recognize when weighing the baby is an appropriate activity to undertake.

You may wonder why it is important to even debate this issue. What could possibly be the problem with weighing the baby at every visit, for example? Some of the issues to consider include using professional judgment and promoting parental confidence.

Using professional judgment

There is a need to move away from ritualistic practice. Much midwifery education encourages the student to develop critical thinking skills and an ability to make decisions based on the best available evidence. Faced with caring for individual women, in a range of settings, midwives need to be able to judge the most appropriate course of action in each case. For example, a piece of research may suggest that weighing the baby every week is sufficient to detect adequate growth. However, the student needs to ask, 'Where was this research undertaken? Was a range of social groups, educational levels and ages represented? Was there a high level of continuity of care? Were both multiparous and primiparous women included? Were all the babies born at full term and 'normal' birthweights?'

Activity

Define the terms 'light for gestational age', 'low birthweight' and 'very low birthweight'?

What action would a midwife take if a baby had not regained its birthweight by age 10 days?

Promoting parental confidence

Parents need to be given tools to assess whether their baby is thriving other than waiting for the midwife or health visitor to come along with her scales. If the baby is demanding feeds, taking them well and producing at least six wet nappies per 24 hours, then it is likely to be thriving. Babies who are losing weight begin to develop loose skin, particularly noticeable in the legs.

If there is any question about whether a baby is losing too much weight, it should be weighed (naked or in a dry nappy), taking note if the baby has recently fed. A plan should be made to re-weigh the baby using the same scales and conditions if possible. When the same midwife is visiting a family she is much more likely to pick up whether or not the baby appears to be losing weight. When visiting a baby who appears to be losing weight for the first time, it becomes more important to ask questions about the baby's behaviour and feeding patterns in order to assess the situation.

Involving the partner

Families are complex social phenomena and their composition variable, for example: a traditional married couple and their biological children or a same sex partnership with children conceived by introfertilization. In 2006 (Office for National Statistics 2008) 75% of families with dependent children were headed by a couple who were cohabiting or married and approximately 22% were lone mothers and 3% lone fathers. It is not the midwife's place to judge which situation is the most appropriate but to support the family to adjust to their own unique circumstances.

Around the time of the baby's birth, many partners take time off work to support the mother and get to know their new baby. Research has shown that there are many advantages to fathers being involved in the care of their baby. For example, those dads who undertake a lot of care bond with their baby more quickly and enjoy being a parent more than those

who do not (Barclay & Lupton 1999). Father involvement is also linked with less depression in mothers (Fisher et al 1999). The midwife is ideally placed to facilitate partner involvement in baby care and provide praise and encouragement for the involvement she either sees or hears reported by the mother.

Neonatal screening test

Parents need information about the neonatal screening test that is offered to all babies at approximately 1 week of age. Although all health authorities offer neonatal screening, there are still some differences between them in terms of the conditions that are screened for. The midwife must have knowledge of the tests undertaken in her area and be able to counsel parents about the nature of the diseases screened for, their incidence and possible treatment. For details regarding the procedure, refer to *Midwifery Essentials: basics* (Baston et al 2009).

Contraception

Women should be reminded that it is possible for them to get pregnant again before their periods resume (normally within three to six weeks, unless breastfeeding). Although sex may be the furthest thought from their mind in the first few days after the birth, they should be prepared for the likelihood that this aspect of their lives will resume in the not too distant future. They will need advice specific to their individual needs, and this issue is discussed in further detail in Chapter 9.

Transfer to the care of the health visitor

The NSF (2004) recommended that midwives and health visitors should work closely together, and that when the mother's post-birth needs have been addressed her care can be transferred to the health visitor. When handover of care from midwife to health visitor takes place, it is essential that effective liaison takes place between the two agencies. It has been reported that this is a difficult transition for some women (Singh & Newburn 2001). Community midwives and health visitors may be attached to the same GP practice, but this is not always the case, with some having caseloads based on a geographical location rather than on GP population.

The community midwife will inform the woman when to expect a visit from her health visitor, depending on local arrangements. The health visitor has usually made a visit during the pregnancy or taken part in preparation for parenthood classes, so that the woman knows who she is and has some understanding of her role. The priorities for health visitors vary depending on the area in which they work, so midwives need to be familiar with the focus of care from their local health visitor.

A small study (Hunter 2004) aimed at first-time couples' views of the support provided by community midwives during postnatal visits highlights some important issues – for a critical appraisal of this paper see Wray (2004). One of the themes that emerged was that women wished to have their care handed over to the health visitor later. They also wanted more carer continuity and more practical support, particularly with breastfeeding. Another study (Young 2008) showed that first-time mothers would also value information about emotional and relationship changes and more opportunities for peer support.

Reflection on trigger

Look back on the trigger scenario.

Vanessa had been in hospital for two days following the birth of her first child by ventouse extraction. She returned home to a sink full of dirty dishes, over-flowing bins and an empty fridge. Her partner went out again to return the car he had borrowed from his mate. She slumped onto the sofa holding her sleeping daughter and closed her eyes.

Now that you are familiar with postnatal care in the community you should have insight into how the scenario relates to the evidence about this aspect of the midwife's role. The jigsaw model will now be used to explore the trigger scenario in more depth.

Effective communication

Efficient communication between midwives is particularly important when a woman is transferred from one service to another. The midwife in the community will need an accurate account of what has happened to the woman during her hospital stay in order to tailor the care she subsequently offers. The midwife will also need to be able to communicate effectively with the woman and her family as she works with them to provide the support they need. Questions that arise from the scenario might include: Does Vanessa know who she can contact for advice and support? What information does the community midwife receive from the hospital about Vanessa's birth experience? Is this in a format that is accessible to Vanessa? What written information is given to women by the community midwife? Is this information in the literature discussed with the woman?

Woman-centred care

Postnatal care should be planned in accordance with the woman's needs and individual circumstances. However, being able to be flexible about how care is provided is also dependent on there being a range of services on offer. Where possible, women should be offered choices about the timing and content of the care they receive. Care should reflect the needs of the woman rather than the service provider. Questions that arise from the scenario might include: At a postnatal visit, how are decisions made about when Vanessa is next seen by her community midwife? How are individual plans of care formulated where you work? Where are they documented? Are they flexible and responsive to individual circumstances?

Using best evidence

It is a professional requirement to base midwifery care on the best available evidence (NMC 2008). However, many aspects of care have become routine and undertaken because 'that is how we do it here'. Questions that arise from the scenario might include: What mechanisms are there for midwives to challenge custom and practice where you work? Are there any discussion groups or journal clubs that encourage midwives to discuss practice in the light of the research available? How do we know that one particular way of doing something is better than another? What data are routinely gathered from community midwifery care that provide feedback about the effectiveness of the services on offer?

Professional and legal issues

One of the key 'activities of a midwife' (NMC 2004:36) is to 'care for and monitor the progress of the mother in the postnatal period' (op cit: 37) with the purpose of enabling the woman to mother her baby with confidence, knowledge and skill. The midwife has a duty of care to the woman and should work towards making the most of her contact with her, always acting in her best interests. Questions that arise from the scenario might include: What continuing professional development opportunities are available to midwives to enable them to constantly update their knowledge and skills? How are midwives reminded of their professional and legal accountability? Who audits the quality of community midwives postnatal record keeping? What action might be taken as a result of an audit of midwifery records?

Team working

Working with others to achieve the best possible outcomes for women and their babies does not just include the multi-professional team but may also include working with her family and friends where appropriate. Some women are extremely well supported after the birth of their baby, but others may be living with considerable challenges like Vanessa, for example, with extreme poverty of financial and social support. Also, just because a woman has her mother coming to stay, does not necessarily mean that she can rest and relax. Midwives need to understand not only what support a woman has, but the nature of that input and how it is perceived by the woman. Questions that arise from the scenario might include: What is Vanessa's support network? Is her partner taking time off work? How much help does he provide with domestic duties? Will he share baby care responsibilities with Vanessa? What practical advice can the midwife offer Vanessa to help her cope with the turmoil she faces? If Vanessa was a non-English speaking immigrant, what support services are available to enhance care provision?

Clinical dexterity

The midwife uses a range of clinical skills throughout the postnatal period. For example, s/he may need to take out stitches or palpate the woman's abdomen. She will weigh babies and undertake neonatal screening. She will need to undertake these skills with poise and dexterity to maintain the woman's confidence in her competence as a midwife. The midwife must ensure that her body language does not disclose any feelings of distaste for Vanessa's home circumstances. Questions that arise from the scenario might include: How will the midwife undertake her clinical role within this chaotic environment? How does the midwife learn to use her clinical skills in a range of settings? What equipment does the community midwife carry in her car? How does the midwife keep up-to-date with adult and neonatal resuscitation?

Models of care

Providing care that is accessible to all women is a challenge for maternity services. For some women, the traditional model of home visiting will suit them well. However, for others who want to be more flexible in terms of when and how they see the community midwife, a drop-in service or community clinic provides them with an alternative that may be more appropriate to their needs. Questions that arise from the scenario might include: If Vanessa attended a drop-in clinic for her postnatal care, how would the community midwife have insight into her personal circumstances? What services are available to women in the locality where you work? Are these options offered to all women? Do women where you work have a named community midwife that they have developed a relationship with in the antenatal period? What are the advantages and disadvantages of the different models of providing postnatal care?

Safe environment

The midwife must ensure that when she provides care for a woman or her baby she does not put them in any danger. As a professional the midwife must always work within the limits of her competence and treat people with respect (NMC 2008).

Questions that arise from the scenario might include: What risks does the environment that Vanessa has come home to pose to her health and that of her baby? Has Vanessa been informed about the risks of falling asleep with her baby on the sofa? How will this information be passed to her partner? What information should the midwife provide Vanessa about protecting her baby against gastroenteritis?

Promotes health

The postnatal period provides an opportunity for the midwife to model good health practices to Vanessa and other members of the family. By the care she provides and the way she undertakes each aspect of it, she is conveying what may be viewed as 'the best way to do it'. It is therefore essential that she ensures that her care is based on the best available evidence and that she does not take short cuts that might be copied by others. Questions that arise from the scenario might include: How might the midwife promote healthy eating to Vanessa during the postnatal period? What action would you take if an adult was smoking in the same room as the baby? How would you encourage Vanessa to do her postnatal exercises? How would you monitor Vanessa's postnatal mental health?

Further scenarios

The following scenarios enable you to consider how specific situations influence the care the midwife provides. Use the jigsaw model to explore the issues raised in each scenario.

Scenario 1

The midwife was just about to leave when she started rummaging in her bag. Bringing out a leaflet the midwife turned to Lindsay and said, 'Oh and it's your baby's blood spot test tomorrow, so read this leaflet and I'll see you after clinic.'

Practice point

Neonatal screening in the first week of life has become a routine part of postnatal care. Carried out by the community midwife, the test involves obtaining samples of the baby's blood (via a heel prick) that are tested in the laboratory for a range of hereditary conditions. The impact of these diseases can be minimized if they are caught early and treatment introduced as soon as possible. They are therefore very important screening tests that can prevent morbidity and enhance the quality of affected babies' lives. Women and their partners need access to information in order to give consent and understand the possible implications of a positive result.

Further questions specific to Scenario 1 include:

1. Had Lindsay received any other information about neonatal screening?
2. Can Lindsay read?
3. What diseases does the screening test look for?
4. What other advice could the midwife have given Lindsay to make the thought of the screening test less traumatic?
5. How does the community midwife document that she has obtained consent from women to undertake the test?
6. What action would the midwife take if Lindsay refused the test?

Scenario 2

Jake was 5 days old. As the midwife undressed him on her knee, she noticed that he had dark discolouration of the skin over his right buttock.

Practice point

It is important that the midwife takes time to look at the baby completely undressed early in the postnatal period. Sometimes the baby is asleep and it may not be appropriate to disturb him, particularly if the parents have had difficulty settling him. However, the midwife needs a baseline from which the baby's future condition can be judged, so the earlier the baby is examined the better. Discolouration of the skin could be related to child abuse or a birth mark and should be taken seriously.

Further questions specific to Scenario 2 include:

1. Has the baby been undressed by the midwife before?
2. Is there any documentation from the hospital that alerts the midwife that a birth mark was discovered at birth?
3. How should the parents be approached about the mark?
4. What other indications might lead the midwife to suspect child abuse?
5. What action should the midwife take if she suspects that the baby may have been abused?
6. What are the phases of discoloration of a bruise?

Conclusion

Women value the continuity of care provided by the midwife in the postnatal period. It is a privilege to care for women throughout pregnancy and then after the birth at this special time in their lives. Midwifery care can make a difference to how a woman experiences and remembers her baby's first weeks. There is considerable potential to develop and extend this care to help women and their families gain confidence and develop their parenting skills.

Resources

Child protection guidance for senior nurses, health visitors, midwives and their managers. http://www.dh.gov.uk/en/Publicationsandstatistics/Publications/PublicationsPolicyAndGuidance/DH_4017211.

Fatherhood Institute: http://www.fatherhoodinstitute.org/.

Foundation for the Study of Infant Death: http://www.sids.org.uk/.

General Household survey overview. http://www.statistics.gov.uk/

downloads/theme_compendia/GHS06/GHS2006overview.pdf.

National Society for the Prevention of Cruelty to Children (NSPCC): http://www.nspcc.org.uk/HelpAndAdvice/WhatChildAbuse/whatischildabuse_wda36500.html.

Reduce the Risk of Cot Death leaflet for parents: http://www.fsid.org.uk/editpics/404-1.pdf.

UK newborn screening centre: http://www.newbornscreening-bloodspot.org.uk/.

References

Barclay L, Lupton D: The experiences of new fatherhood: a sociocultural analysis, *Journal of Advanced Nursing* 29(4):1013–1020, 1999.

Baston H, Durward H: *Examination of the newborn. A practical guide*, London, 2001, Routledge.

Baston H, Hall J, Henley-Einion A: *Midwifery essentials: basics*, Edinburgh, 2009, Elsevier.

Department of Health: *National Service Framework for children, young people and maternity services. Standard 11. Maternity Services*, London, 2004, HMSO.

Department of Health: *Reduce the risk of cot death leaflet for parents*, 2007. Online. Available http://www.fsid.org.uk/editpics/404-1.pdf October 31, 2008.

Fisher K, Mcculloch A, Gershuny J: British fathers and children. *Working paper*, 1999, University of Essex: Institute for Social and Economic Research.

Foundation for the Study of Infant Deaths: *Fact sheet 1. Cot death facts and figures*, 2006a. Online. Available http://www.fsid.org.uk/editpics/1553-1.pdf October 31, 2008.

Foundation for the Study of Infant Deaths: *Smoking and cot death*, 2006b. Online. Available http://www.fsid.org.uk/smoking.html October 31, 2008.

Fraser DM, Cooper MA: *Myles' Textbook for midwives*, Edinburgh, 2003, Elsevier.

Hanss K: Confidence and breastfeeding: a view from the front-line, *MIDIRS Midwifery Digest* 14(3):384–388, 2004.

Hilton T, Messenger M: *The Great Ormond Street Book of baby and child care*, London, 1991, BCA.

Hunter L: The views of women and their partners on the support provided by community midwives during postnatal home visits, *RCM Evidence Based Midwifery* 2(1):20–27, 2004.

Information Centre: *NHS Maternity Statistics, England: 2005-2006*, The Information Centre, 2007.

Johnson R, Taylor W: *Skills for midwifery practice*, ed 3, Edinburgh, 2006, Elsevier.

King's College: *Support workers in maternity services: a national scoping study of NHS Trusts providing maternity care in England 2006*, London, 2007, Florence Nightingale School of Nursing & Midwifery.

McGarvey C, McDonnell M, Chong A, et al: Factors relating to the infant's last sleep environment in suddent infant death syndrome in the Republic of Ireland, *Archives of Disease in Childhood* 88(12):1054–1064, 2003.

National Institute for Health and Clinical Excellence (NICE): *Routine postnatal care of women and their babies*, London, 2006, NICE.

Nursing and Midwifery Council (NMC): *Midwives rules and standards*, London, 2004, NMC.

Nursing and Midwifery Council (NMC): *The Code. Standards of conduct, performance and ethics for nurses and midwives*, London, 2008, NMC.

Office for National Statistics: *General Household Survey 2006*, Newport. Online. Available http://www.statistics.gov.uk/downloads/theme_compendia/GHS06/GHS2006overview.pdf November 1, 2008.

Roberton N: *A manual of normal neonatal care*, London, 1996, Arnold.

Singh D, Newburn M: Postnatal care in the month after birth, *The Practising Midwife* 4(5):22–25, 2001.

United Kingdom Central Council: *Midwives Rules and Code of Practice*, London, 1998, UKCC.

Wray J: Research unwrapped. Postnatal home visits: the parents' views, *The Practising Midwife* 7(9):38–40, 2004.

Wright C, Parkinson K: Postnatal weight loss in term infants: what is 'normal' and do growth charts allow for it?, *Archives of Disease in Childhood* 89(3):F254–F257, 2004.

Young E: Maternal expectations: do they match experience? *Community Practitioner* 81(10):27–30, 2008.

Chapter 8

Emotional wellbeing following birth

Trigger scenario

Sarah gave birth to her first baby, Dominic, three days ago, and is visited by Ella, her midwife. He has started crying again, having just been placed into his crib 10 minutes ago. Sarah sits in bed sobbing, saying, 'I can't do this – I'm no good as a mother!

Introduction

There is a considerable time of adjustment after the arrival of a new baby; a process which continues for many years. Midwives have an important role in helping parents and families in this period of change and adaptation, which includes recognizing when they are not adjusting well. There will be a mixture of emotions over this time, which may have a number of causes. A holistic approach to care that appreciates the continuum between the body-mind-and-spirit (Davis-Floyd 2001), and the 'continuous process from conception through pregnancy, labour, birth and beyond' (NMC 2004:06) will enable a midwife to establish what the cause may be, as well as recognizing if any intervention is required. This process requires midwives to have knowledge of the 'normal' changes within a woman's mental state related to childbirth in order to be able to know when her health is at risk.

The World Health Organization (2008a) defines mental health as:

a state of wellbeing in which every individual realizes his or her own potential, can cope with the normal stresses of life, can work productively and fruitfully, and is able to make a contribution to her or his community.

A further definition of mental health identifies the elements:

- Absence of illness
- Appropriate social behaviour

- Freedom from worry and guilt
- Personal competence and control
- Self-acceptance and self-actualization
- Unification and organization of personality
- Open-mindedness and flexibility. (Swinton 2001:35)

In the postnatal period an important part of a midwifery role will be to help women adapt to being a mother and to 'cope' with her role.

Midwives also have to be aware that what affects the woman may also affect her baby and the support network around her. There is widespread recognition of the impact of postnatal psychological difficulties on the child (Department of Health 2004, WHO 2008b), and researchers have demonstrated the long-term effects on child behaviour (O'Connor et al 2002, Hay et al 2003).

Importantly, the *Saving Mothers' Lives* report (Lewis 2007) demonstrated continued high levels of maternal deaths related to psychological issues following childbirth. Though many deaths occur some time after the baby is born, it is within the midwife's remit to recognize those women who are at risk of severe psychological difficulties, to recognize if there are changes in a woman's mental state and to communicate effectively with other members of the woman's caring team. The NSF (Department of Health 2004) indicates, too, that postnatal care should be long term in order to be able to recognize and act on the more serious postnatal health issues that do not arise until some time after the birth.

The aim of this chapter is to consider some of the emotional issues that may affect a woman, her baby and family, in the postnatal period, and to highlight potential psychiatric issues that may arise.

Life change

It should be recognized that for each woman pregnancy and birth bring phenomenal change – physical, emotional, social and spiritual (Hall 2001:64). During the time of transformation to being a mother, development of the maternal 'self' takes place (Rubin 1984). Women have identified this time as the most important learning experience in their lives (Belenky et al 1997). If this process is such a powerful event, it is understandable that from an emotional basis there will need to be a time of adjustment during the whole continuum. The emotions that are experienced may alter throughout the duration of the pregnancy, and will probably be different for each pregnancy the woman experiences (Baston 2003).

Activity

Consider what adjustment issues might face a very young or older mother, a mother who has been employed, or a woman with an unwell infant.

Think about the advice you would give a woman antenatally to help her maximize her postnatal health.

Providing individualized, woman-centred care that can be adapted to individual needs may help ensure the most appropriate care for that woman. Building up a relationship with the woman in the antenatal period and caring for her postnatally makes it easier for carers to recognize what is normal for that particular woman and if there are any physical, emotional or social changes that might have an effect on her wellbeing. This is the ideal situation, and the *Maternity Matters* report stipulates that:

Women and their partners will be supported by a midwife they know and trust before and after birth.

(Department of Health 2007:09)

Many women may have pre-existing mental health issues prior to pregnancy, (Boxes 8.1 & 8.2) and this knowledge should inform how midwives plan care, involving the woman and the multi-disciplinary team (Price 2004).

Box 8.1 Common mental health disorders (WHO 2004)

- Anxiety disorders
- Depression
- Panic disorders
- Post-traumatic stress disorder
- Phobia
- Obsessive-compulsive disorder
- Adjustment disorder
- Addiction
- Eating disorders

Recognition also needs to be given to the partner, who is adapting psychologically to a new role as well as coping with a woman who is recovering physically from pregnancy and birth. Partners have said they felt 'left out' after the birth of a baby, and midwives should remember to ask how the partner is feeling and allow them time to communicate their feelings. Aiming to build a relationship with the partner in the antenatal period is beneficial to the midwife noting changes in behaviour in the partner after the baby is born.

Box 8.2 More serious mental health disorders (Weeks 2007)

- Affective disorders
- Schizophrenia

Physical issues

In order to provide psychological care midwives should recognize the impact of the changes to a woman's body. For example, following birth the hormones that have been circulating and supporting the maintenance of the baby will no longer be required to the same levels, and they drop at different speeds. The need for the body to establish hormonal stability may have an effect on the emotional state of the woman.

Body image

Issues relating to the woman's altered body image will have taken place during her pregnancy (Price 1993, Baston & Hall 2009) which is linked to self-esteem (Lavender 2007). The type of birth she experienced may have had an effect on the way she feels about herself postnatally. Any physical trauma the woman has endured should not be decried as trivial but treated with extreme sensitivity (Way 1996). She may want to achieve her previous weight or 'flat' abdominal muscles. The strength of these desires may influence her behaviour in the postnatal period, and frustration may develop if she is unable to achieve her personal goals. Perceptions may also be influenced by the cultural 'norm' for the woman (Boyington et al 2007). Furthermore, her feelings about her body may have an influence on her choice of feeding method, with women who feel more dissatisfaction with their body being less likely to choose breastfeeding (Foster et al 1996). Negative views of breasts as sexual objects or fears about touch may also have an effect on her views about feeding her baby (Hall 1997). In addition, change in libido and her perception of her body may have a positive or a negative effect on her sexual relationship with her partner (Snellen 2006).

Lack of sleep

A key issue affecting maternal (and partner) mental health is sleep deprivation (Bozoky & Corwin 2002). This may be heightened in the initial postnatal period and be related to an altered pattern in REM sleep, leading to greater fatigue (Lee et al 2000). This may be worsened in women who are recovering from long and exhausting labours that have resulted in traumatic or surgical birth. Busy postnatal wards, which include large numbers of postnatal mothers, are not the most ideal places for women to achieve restful sleep (Sherr 1995).

Midwives need to consider how postnatal hospital care can be adapted to enable a postnatal woman to rest, which includes adapting 'routine' care to fit in with opportunity for sleep. This can be a challenge where certain 'tasks' are seen to need to be achieved over a shift pattern. However, recognition that sleep and rest are part of healing and restoration and vital to the mental wellbeing of a postnatal woman is important. Taking steps to lower noise levels on wards at all times, especially at night, are essential. This could include the type of shoes midwives choose to wear, and the way conversations are conducted, as well as the levels at which televisions or radios are played. The use of noisy equipment should be kept to a minimum, and reduction of light level is essential at night. Sensitive communication with visitors is important, especially in situations where relatives have travelled long distances. Provision of written information to partners of the need for postnatal rest is valuable, and could be used to pass on to other relatives.

Advice regarding gaining rest during the baby's sleep times at home should also be given. The midwife should be especially aware of those women who have limited social support or other children to care for, as they may have fewer opportunities to sleep when the baby is resting.

Activity

Consider your postnatal areas of working.

Think about how care can be adapted to ensure adequate sleep is promoted.

The NICE guideline of postnatal care (2006:95) indicates that midwives should encourage women to:

help look after their mental health by looking after themselves. This includes taking gentle exercise, taking time to rest, getting help with caring for the baby, talking to someone about their feelings and ensuring they can access social support networks.

Spiritual issues

The Royal College of Psychiatrists highlight the importance of the spiritual dimension in relation to mental wellbeing (Royal College of Psychiatrists 2006). Spiritual care could lead to:

- improved self-control, self-esteem and confidence

- faster and easier recovery, achieved through both promoting the healthy grieving of loss and maximizing personal potential
- improved relationships – with self, others and with God/creation/nature
- a new sense of meaning, resulting in reawakening of hope and peace of mind, enabling people to accept and live with problems not yet resolved. (Royal College of Psychiatrists 2006)

During the postnatal period midwives can help to promote women's self-esteem and sense of meaning and purpose by recognizing the transformative nature of birth. Spiritual and religious beliefs may have become more significant during pregnancy, with these providing a source of coping with stressful situations (Carver & Ward 2007, Jesse et al 2007, Price et al 2007). Midwives in the community should be aware of the religious communities in their area and it may be beneficial to establish what postnatal support may be available for information and referral purposes (Hall 2001).

'Baby blues'

Women will commonly experience emotional feelings following the birth of their babies. Box 8.3 indicates the timing of these experiences after birth. The 'blues' is thought to be a transient state of heightened emotional reactivity which is said to affect about 70% of postnatal women. It may last up to 10 days following birth (Ussher 2004). The intensity of the symptoms a woman experiences will be individual to her and may be linked to hormonal imbalances, psychological effects or social phenomena (Miller 2002, Ussher 2004). The signs and symptoms, illustrated in Box 8.4, are varied.

Women who experience the blues are more likely to progress to a postnatal depressive condition (Beck et al 1992, Henshaw et al 2004).

Box 8.3 Timing of depression following childbirth (Ussher 2004: 109)

- 'The blues': weeping and anxiety occurring between 2 and 10 days following birth. Transitory.
- Depression and anxiety on arriving home with a new baby. Lasts a week or two.
- Depressed moods with good and bad days. Up to three months after birth.
- Clinical depression. Enduring symptoms such as anxiety, sleep and appetite disturbance.

Box 8.4 Signs and symptoms of 'baby blues'

- Mood swings
- Irritability
- Tearfulness
- Confusion
- Forgetfulness
- Hostility
- Heightened response to stimuli

Activity

Consider how a midwife might respond when a woman is showing symptoms of 'baby blues'.

What advice and support could she give to the woman's partner?

National guidance from NICE (2006) indicates midwives should ask women at each postnatal contact:

what family and social support they have and their usual coping strategies for dealing with day to day matters

(NICE 2006:95)

The woman and her family should also be:

encouraged to tell their healthcare professional about any changes in mood, emotional state and behaviour that are outside of the woman's normal pattern

(NICE 2006:95)

Further it is advised that:

at 10–14 days after birth, all women should be asked about resolution of symptoms of baby blues (for example, tearfulness, feelings of anxiety and low mood). If symptoms have not resolved, the woman should be assessed for postnatal depression, and if symptoms persist, further evaluated

(NICE 2006:95)

Though midwives may have handed over care to a community practitioner by this time, it indicates that adequate information about the severity and length of the time should be communicated at handover in order for further assessment to be made.

Postnatal depressive conditions

There has been some debate in recent years as to whether postnatal depressive conditions are pathological illnesses or an 'understandable response to the difficulties of motherhood' (Ussher 2004). The conditions most described are non-psychotic postnatal depression or postnatal psychosis (Miller 2002, Brockington 2004). However, women may also present with other conditions such as extreme anxiety, maternal/child relationship disorders, obsessive behaviours, substance misuse, eating disorders or post traumatic stress disorder (PTSD). Awareness of these conditions is important in relation to the wellbeing of the mother (Lewis 2007) and the partner (Goodman 2004) but also to the potential long-term wellbeing of the child (Martins & Gaffan 2000, Hay et al 2003, Murray et al 2003, Luoma et al 2004).

Non-psychotic postnatal depression

Prevalence

As indicated in Box 8.3, most women will experience some episodes of emotional fluctuations following birth.

Our concern here is the issue of clinical depression, a serious condition with symptoms that can present at any time from 4 weeks to 1 year after birth. It appears that the occurrence of depression in postnatal women is comparable to the rates in all women. However, Cox et al (1993) showed a rate of depression in the first month after childbirth that was three times the average monthly incidence in non-childbearing women. O'Hara & Swain's (1996) meta-analysis of studies found the incidence of postnatal depression to be 12–13% though this may be as high as 20% (Royal College of Midwives 2007). Importantly, a link has been demonstrated to antenatal depression (Evans et al 2001, Stowe et al 2005), indicating that midwives should be particularly aware of women with depressive disorders during pregnancy.

Women at risk

In a study carried out in the 1980s, Ball (1994) demonstrated that there were certain factors in women's ability to cope with motherhood (Box 8.5). This indicates that midwives should be

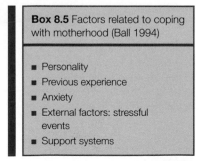

Box 8.5 Factors related to coping with motherhood (Ball 1994)

- Personality
- Previous experience
- Anxiety
- External factors: stressful events
- Support systems

able to identify those more at risk of not being able to cope because of a lack of support, increased levels of stress or higher levels of anxiety in pregnancy.

Women who are thought to be more at risk of depressive illness following birth are listed in Box 8.6.

> **Box 8.6** Risk factors for postnatal depression (Kennedy et al 2002)
>
> - Prior history of depressive illness before or during pregnancy
> - Childcare stress
> - Life stress
> - Lack of social support
> - Prenatal anxiety
> - Maternity blues
> - Relationship dissatisfaction
> - Low self-esteem
> - Low socio-economic status
> - Single
> - Unplanned or undesired pregnancy

There may be genetic factors related to the development of postnatal depression in some cases (Forty et al 2006). One study (McMahon et al 2005) suggests that a woman's childhood, as well as any current relationship difficulties, may have an effect on the duration of depression. It is important to take a careful antenatal and family history in order to be able to recognize those women at risk after the birth. Also, midwives should be increasingly aware of any social needs a woman may have.

Activity

Consider how midwives find out about a woman's family history.

Find out how midwives in your area use identified risk factors to adapt the care they give to women in the postnatal period.

Midwives care

The experience of depression is varied and includes a range of symptoms (Box 8.7).

> **Box 8.7** Signs and symptoms of depressive conditions (Kennedy et al 2002)
>
> - Feeling a failure as a mother
> - Feelings of panic
> - Loss of appetite
> - Fear of hurting yourself or your baby
> - Feeling guilty
> - Feelings of anxiousness and insecurity
> - Feeling overwhelmed
> - Crying a lot
> - Feeling you are not normal or real anymore
> - Difficulty sleeping
> - Angry – feeling you might explode
> - Feeling lonely
> - Unable to make decisions
> - Inability to concentrate or focus
> - Thinking the baby might be better off without you

If a midwife has had the opportunity to develop a relationship with the woman prior to birth, she may be able to identify relatively quickly if there is a change in the woman's behaviour or personality. The woman may also feel more comfortable about sharing her anxieties or concerns about herself. Bick et al (2002) helpfully provide guidelines for assessing women's mental wellbeing (Box 8.8). Midwives should follow local pathways of care, where these are available.

Box 8.8 Summary guideline: depression and other psychological morbidity (Bick et al 2002:143–144)

Initial assessment

- Ask how the woman is feeling: is she anxious, disappointed with the baby/maternal experience, unable to sleep?
- Ask her about support from her partner, relatives, friends
- Be especially aware if there is a history of psychiatric illness, her relationship with her partner is difficult or she is unsupported, or if what appeared to be the 'blues' does not resolve.

Immediate referral to GP required if:

- Woman showing symptoms of puerperal psychosis
- Woman whom midwife considers to be at risk of suicide or child abuse.

What to do if a woman shows symptoms of depression:

- If concerned that a woman may be depressed, discuss this and refer to GP and inform health visitor.
- Encourage support of partner (and/or close relative or friend) in caring for baby.
- Ensure that the woman knows how to contact the midwife and/or health visitor at any time.
- Offer self-help and support group literature.
- If, at any time, the midwife suspects the existence of other psychological morbidity, such as severe anxiety disorders or stress reactions, the woman should be referred to her GP.

The NICE antenatal and postnatal mental health guideline (NICE 2007:09) recommends that women should be asked at around 4–6 weeks and 3–4 months postnatally:

- During the past month, have you often been bothered by feeling down, depressed or hopeless?
- During the past month, have you often been bothered by having little interest or pleasure in doing things?

A third question should then be considered if the woman answers 'yes' to either of the initial questions: Is this something you feel you need or want help with?

They also indicate that further research needs to be carried out on whether this is a valid tool for midwives and health visitors (NICE 2007:28).

Other scales have been devised as tools to screen for those women who are at risk of depressive disorders, that assess their condition through answers to a questionnaire. Commonly, the Edinburgh postnatal depression scale (EPDS) (Cox et al 1987) is used, though others use the Beck postpartum depression screening scale (PDSS) (Beck & Gable 2001). In one study, non-respondents to the EPDS demonstrated higher levels of postnatal depression (George & Elliott 2004). This indicates that an element of caution needs to be taken when women do not respond.

Activity

Identify which depression scale is used in your locality.

Find out who administers the questionnaire, when and how.

Treatment

Several different treatments for postnatal depression are advocated, and may vary according to the diagnosis of the condition, choice of the woman, availability of the treatment and the person making the diagnosis (Boath & Henshaw 2003, NICE 2007). In recent years, a more holistic approach to avoid medication has been advocated (Box 8.9;

Kennedy et al 2002, Miller 2002, Ray & Hodnett 2004).

A Cochrane review (Dennis & Hodnett 2007) has shown that, in the short term, psychosocial and psychological interventions may be an effective measure in helping women with postnatal depression. NICE recommend (NICE 2007) a 'stepped approach' to care:

- Self-help strategies
- Non-directive counselling
- Brief cognitive behavioural therapy
- Interpersonal psychotherapy.

If a woman declines the psychological therapy, if it does not work or if she has previously had a history of severe depression then treatment with antidepressants is suggested. Further evidence has shown that there may be a link with partner depression and the woman being depressed (Goodman 2004). Therefore, the midwife should be aware if there is an issue with the partner being unwell in order to care effectively for the woman and her baby. Alternative therapies may also be useful: practising infant massage (Onozawa

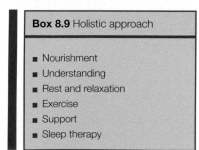

Box 8.9 Holistic approach

- Nourishment
- Understanding
- Rest and relaxation
- Exercise
- Support
- Sleep therapy

Activity

Access the NICE guideline for antenatal and postnatal mental health:

http://www.nice.org.uk/guidance/index.jsp?action=download&o=30431 and look at the different forms of drug therapy that is availabe.

Find out about St John's Wort, and in what way it is used to treat depression.

et al 2001) has also been shown to benefit both the mother's level of depression and interaction with the infant.

Postnatal psychosis

The most severe form of mental illness following birth is termed postnatal psychosis though there is some concern about making a distinctive diagnosis (NICE 2007). It is a psychiatric emergency which occurs within three weeks of the birth (Miller 2002), sometimes as early as one to two days after the baby is born (Cantwell & Cox 2003).

The term describes a group of illnesses that manifest by delusions and hallucinations (Brockington 2004). It is thought to affect 1–2 per 1000 births (Cantwell & Cox 2003). Those women who are most at risk have had a personal history of affective psychosis, a previous history of puerperal psychosis or a close relation with affective psychosis (Cantwell & Cox 2003, Brockington 2004). Women who present with psychotic depression can appear

well initially, but then may become profoundly depressed or psychotic very quickly (Miller 2002). Potential symptoms are listed in Table 8.1.

Care and treatment

Immediate care of the mother, infant and her family will involve ensuring safety. Midwives who have concerns about a women should refer to medical help as soon as possible. Referral to psychiatric services should be rapid, and most women will require hospital admission. Ideally, the mother and baby should be kept together, but this will depend on the availability of a mother and baby unit in the local psychiatric hospital. The midwife's role will involve supporting the family during the admission and continuing to provide postnatal care in hospital. The care will involve restoration of the woman's self-confidence, enabling her to build a relationship with the infant and develop mothering skills. A combination of antipsychotic, antidepressive and mood-regulator drugs

Table 8.1 Differential symptoms of postnatal depression, psychosis and mania

Depressive	Manic	Psychotic
Frequent tearfulness	Overactivity	Delusions
Sadness	Elated	Visual or auditory
Suicidal ideas	Over-talkative	Hallucinations
Poor appetite	Restlessness	Intrusive thoughts
Poor sleep	Irritability	Unusual beliefs
Poor concentration	Disorientation in time, place, person	Non-recognition and non-identification of those around

will be used. Electroconvulsive therapy may also be used (Cantwell & Cox 2003, Brockington 2004). Care should also be given to the partner and family members, who may be quite shocked by the experience. Also, staff and students who have been involved should be supported effectively as this may be a rare and traumatic occurrence (Price 2004).

Reflection on trigger

Look back on the trigger scenario.

Sarah gave birth to her first baby, Dominic, three days ago, and is visited by Ella her midwife. He has started crying again, having just been placed into his crib 10 minutes ago. Sarah sits in bed sobbing, saying, 'I can't do this – I'm no good as a mother!'

The scenario describes an event in the postnatal period that could have taken place in any situation. Now that you are familiar with the issues around emotional wellbeing in the postnatal period you should have insight into how the scenario relates to current midwifery practice. The jigsaw model will now be used to explore the trigger scenario in more depth.

Effective communication

In the postnatal period communication skills are vital, especially when there are concerns about a woman's mental wellbeing. Careful observation of body language and behaviour around the baby are important, as well as discussion with the family. Questions that could be asked are: Has Ella previously

developed a relationship with Sarah? Is her behaviour different? What questions could be asked about Sarah's feelings? What clues may be obtained from her responses and physical behaviour? How should the discussion be recorded?

Woman-centred care

This involves recognition of Sarah as an individual and aiming to provide sensitive care that ensures she is central to all decision-making about her care. It is important that care is informed by an awareness of Sarah's family and previous medical history. Questions that could be asked are: Is this a 'routine' visit by Ella or planned because of a request or concern? Has Sarah been included in the plan for her care? Does she have a partner or family included in her support? What has been her experience, of pregnancy, labour and postnatal care so far?

Using best evidence

Ella needs to use the best evidence available to make decisions about what is happening to Sarah and her baby and the next aspects of her care. An understanding of the evidence around perinatal mental health treatment will enable Ella to answer questions that Sarah and her partner might have about how she is feeling. Questions that could be asked are: What will she ask to establish what Sarah is experiencing? What is the evidence about causes and diagnosis of postnatal mental health issues? What evidence is available about care and treatment? What national guidance is available to establish the most appropriate care and support?

Professional and legal issues

Midwives should always practise within the framework of professional rules and the legal system. Ella should act in Sarah's best interests at all times and gain consent for any actions she might plan to take. Questions that could be asked are: Is Ella trained appropriately to understand postnatal mental health issues? Is she confident in the care of women in the postnatal period? How do the rules of practice and the NMC Code guide in the care of women with emotional or mental health needs? Is there national or professional guidance available?

Team working

It is not clear in this scenario if this is taking place in a hospital or community setting. However, in all situations midwives work in a service where there are other midwives and health professionals to provide support if required. Questions that could be asked are: Are the needs of Sarah enough to require inclusion of other health professionals? If so, who will this be? How will this referral take place? Where will information be recorded for other health professionals to access? What opportunities are there for interprofessional learning around perinatal health issues?

Clinical dexterity

In this situation in relation to emotional issues, clinical skills may not usually be required. However, if the midwife needs to carry out any tests following on from the discussion, she should use sensitivity and gentleness, performing her care with dexterity. Questions that could arise are: Does Ella need to make any clinical assessments in relation to Sarah's care? Is this the appropriate time to carry out these assessments? How might Sarah's physical progress impact on how she is feeling? What observations should Ella perform to assess Sarah's physical health?

Models of care

A variety of models of midwifery care are practised in the UK. How care is organized may have a positive or negative effect on the emotional wellbeing of some women. In this situation, questions that could be raised are: Does Ella work in a team of colleagues who aim to provide continuity through from pregnancy into the postnatal period? Would continuity of postnatal care be beneficial in this situation? Is home-based care more beneficial in this situation? If so, why would this be? Are there other professional groups involved in the provision of the care Ella is giving?

Safe environment

All midwifery care should be carried out in a safe environment, for the woman, her family members and also for the midwife. The unpredictability of mental health issues means that midwives should be vigilant to ensure safety is maintained, both for the mother, but also for the baby. Questions that could be asked about this scenario are: Is Sarah currently in a safe environment or are there reasons to believe she may be putting herself or her baby and family at risk? Is Ella safe in visiting Sarah as a lone professional?

If the environment is not considered safe whom should Ella contact for assistance?

Promotes health

The postnatal period provides many opportunities for midwives to promote the emotional health of a woman, her family and the community in which they work. In this scenario questions that could be asked to ensure that the woman's care promotes health include: Does the environment where Sarah is living promote her mental wellbeing? Are there issues in her situation that are damaging her health? Are there ways Ella could promote Sarah's emotional health at this time? What advice might Ella offer other members of Sarah's support network that might enhance how she is feeling?

Further scenarios

The following scenarios enable you to consider how specific situations influence the care the midwife provides. Use the jigsaw model to explore the issues raised in each situation.

Scenario 1

Maria is 10 days post birth of her second baby. Caroline has come to visit her at home to transfer them to the care of the Health Visitor. Following Maria's previous birth she was diagnosed with severe postnatal depression.

Practice point

Women who have had a previous episode of depression following birth are susceptible to this again following subsequent births. Midwifery care will involve careful observation and awareness of factors that may increase her chances of the condition. Further she should also ensure information is given to the woman and her family about signs of when to ask for help. Careful documentation may also alert other professionals to the condition.

Questions that could be asked in the care of Maria are:

1. How did Maria experience depression after her last birth?
2. What were the signs and symptoms?
3. What are her fears in this situation?
4. What are the fears of her partner?
5. What questions may Caroline ask?
6. What information/guidance may she give to Maria and her family?
7. Are there local support groups available?
8. What information will Caroline give her Health Visitor/GP?

Scenario 2

Dawn is a midwife on a postnatal ward. A baby is crying continuously and she walks into a four bed bay to find the baby of one day old has been left alone in the crib. One of the other mothers says they have seen her mother, Tina, walking down the ward. At that moment the ward phone rings and a porter says they have prevented a woman called Tina in a dressing gown from trying to leave the building. Dawn goes to fetch her to find Tina is saying strange sentences repetitively. She does not acknowledge Dawn at all.

Practice point

Psychotic behaviour post birth can happen very suddenly and may manifest in different ways. It is not a midwife's responsibility to diagnose a serious mental condition but to ensure referral to the appropriate professional is speedy. She should also ensure the safety of both the mother and the baby until help is available.

Questions that may be asked in this situation are:

1. What ways will Dawn try to communicate with Tina to establish her needs?
2. What questions may she ask and what observations will she carry out?
3. What may Tina be experiencing?
4. How will Dawn consider the needs of the other women on the ward?
5. How will the needs of the baby be met?
6. Who will Dawn contact for assistance?
7. What documentation may be completed?

8. How will Tina be best cared for?
9. What will be the involvement of the family in this situation?

Conclusion

Midwives have a clear role to play in the identification of those women at risk of postnatal mental illness. The danger of labelling conditions as psychiatric in origin that may turn out to have a physical source should be noted (Lewis 2007). Furthermore, there should be clear communication pathways between community services and mental health services to ensure that effective treatment is provided (Lewis 2007). It has been shown that intensive postnatal support by midwives and health visitors is of benefit to women (Dennis & Creedy 2004). The indication is that providers of postnatal services should invest in evidence-based care to support women and their families (Department of Health 2004).

Resources

Association for postnatal illness: www.apni.org/pndleaflet.htm.

Mental Health Foundation: http://www.mentalhealth.org.uk/information/mental-health-a-z/postnatal-depression/.

Mind: http://www.mind.org.uk/Information/Booklets/Understanding/Understanding + postnatal + depression.htm.

National Collaborating Centre for Mental Health: *Antenatal and postnatal mental health. The NICE guideline*

on clinical management and service guidance: http://www.nice.org.uk/guidance/index.jsp?action=download&o=30431, London, 2007, NICE.

NHS Direct: Postnatal depression. http://www.nhsdirect.nhs.uk/articles/article.aspx?articleId=429.

Price SA, editor: *Mental health in pregnancy and childbirth*, Churchill Livingstone, 2007, Edinburgh.

Royal College of Psychiatrists: http://www.rcpsych.ac.uk/.

References

Ball JA: *Reactions to motherhood*, ed 2, Books for Midwives Press, 1994, Cheshire.

Baston H: Antenatal care – monitoring maternal well-being, *The Practising Midwife* 6(3):32–35, 2003.

Baston H, Hall J: *Midwifery essentials: antenatal*, Edinburgh, 2009, Elsevier.

Beck CT, Gable RK: Further validation of the postpartum depression screening scale, *Nursing Research* 50(30):155–164, 2001.

Beck C, Reynolds MA, Rutowski P: Maternity blues and postpartum depression, *Journal of Obstetric, Gynecologic and Neonatal Nursing* 21(4):287–293, 1992.

Belenky MF, Clinchy BM, Goldberger NR, et al: *Women's way of knowing*, 10th anniversary edn, New York, 1997, Basic Books.

Bick D, MacArthur C, Knowles H, et al: *Postnatal care: evidence and guidelines for management*, Edinburgh, 2002, Churchill Livingstone.

Boath E, Henshaw C: The treatment of postnatal depression: a comprehensive literature review, *Journal of Reproductive and Infant Psychology* 19(30):215–248, 2003.

Boyington J, Johnson A, Carter-Edwards L: Dissatisfaction with body size among low-income, postpartum black women, *Journal of Obstetric, Gynecologic and Neonatal Nursing* 36(2):144–151, 2007.

Bozoky I, Corwin EJ: Fatigue as a predictor of postpartum depression, *Association of Women's Health, Obstetric and Neonatal Nurses* 31:436–443, 2002.

Brockington I: Postpartum psychiatric disorders, *The Lancet* 363:303–310, 2004.

Cantwell R, Cox JL: Psychiatric disorders in pregnancy and puerperium, *Current Obstetrics & Gynecology* 13:7–13, 2003.

Carver N, Ward B: Spirituality in pregnancy: a diversity of experiences and needs, *British Journal of Midwifery* 15(5):294–296, 2007.

Cox JL, Holden JM, Sagovsky R: Detection of postnatal depression, Development of the 10-item Edinburgh Postnatal Depression Scale. *British Journal of Psychiatry,* 150:782–786, 1987.

Cox JL, Murray D, Chapman G: A controlled study of the onset, duration and prevalence of postnatal depression, *British Journal of Psychiatry* 163:27–31, 1993.

Davis-Floyd R: The technocratic, humanistic, and holistic paradigms of childbirth, *International Journal of Gynecology & Obstetrics* 75:S5–S23, 2001.

Dennis CL, Creedy DK: Psychosocial and psychological interventions for prevention of postpartum depression DOI: 10.1002/14651858.CD001134.pub2, *Cochrane Database of Systematic Reviews* 4(CD001134), 2004.

Dennis CL, Hodnett E: Psychosocial and psychological interventions for treating postpartum depression DOI: 10.1002/14651858.CD006116.pub2, *Cochrane Database of Systematic Reviews* 4(CD006116), 2007.

Department of Health: *Maternity standard. National Service Framework for children, young people and maternity services*, London, 2004, Department of Health.

Department of Health: *Maternity matters: choice, access and continuity of care in a safe service*, London, 2007, Department of Health.

Evans J, Heron J, Francomb H, et al: Cohort study of depressed mood during pregnancy, *British Medical Journal* 323:257–260, 2001.

Forty L, Jones L, MacGregor S, et al: Familiality of postpartum depression in unipolar disorder: results of a family study, *American Journal of Psychiatry* 163:1549–1553, 2006.

Foster SF, Slade P, Wilson K: Body image, maternal fetal attachment and breast feeding, *Journal of Psychosomatic Research* 41(2):181–184, 1996.

George C, Elliott SA: Searching for antenatal predictors of postnatal depressive symptomatology: unexpected findings from a study of obsessive-compulsive personality traits, *Journal of Reproductive and Infant Psychology* 22(1):25–31, 2004.

Goodman JH: Paternal postpartum depression, its relationship to maternal postpartum depression and implications for family health, *Journal of Advanced Nursing* 45(1):26–35, 2004.

Hall J: Breastfeeding and sexuality: societal conflicts and expectations, *British Journal of Midwifery* 5(6):350–354, 1997.

Hall J: *Midwifery mind and spirit: emerging issues of care*, Oxford, 2001, Books for Midwives.

Hay DF, Pawlby S, Angold A, et al: Pathways to violence in the children of mothers who were depressed postpartum, *Developmental Psychology* 39(6):1083–1094, 2003.

Henshaw C, Foreman D, Cox J: Postnatal blues: a risk factor for postnatal depression, *Journal of Psychosomatic Obstetrics & Gynecology* 25(3 & 4): 267–272, 2004. Online. Available http://www.informaworld.com/smpp/title-content=t713634100-db=all-tab=issueslist-branches=25-v25.

Jesse DE, Schoneboom C, Blanchard A: The effect of faith or spirituality in pregnancy: a content analysis, *Journal of Holistic Nursing* 25(3):151–158, 2007.

Kennedy HP, Beck CT, Driscoll JW: A light in the fog: caring for women with postpartum depression, *Journal of Midwifery and Women's Health* 47(5):318–327, 2002.

Lavender V: Body image: change, dissatisfaction and disturbance. In Price S, editor: *Mental health in pregnancy and childbirth*, Edinburgh, 2007, Churchill Livingstone.

Lee KA, Zaffke ME, McEnany G: Parity and sleep patterns during and after pregnancy, *Obstetrics and Gynecology* 95:14–18, 2000.

Lewis GE: The confidential enquiry into maternal and child health (CEMACH). Saving mothers' lives: reviewing maternal deaths to make motherhood safer – 2003–2005. *The 7th report on confidential enquiries into maternal deaths in the United Kingdom*. London, 2007, CEMACH.

Luoma I, et al: A longitudinal study of maternal depressive symptoms, negative expectations and perceptions of child problems, *Child Psychiatry & Human Development* 35(1):37–53, 2004.

Martins C, Gaffan EA: Effects of early maternal depression on patterns of infant-mother attachment: a meta-analytic investigation, *Journal of Child Psychology and Psychiatry* 41(6):737–746, 2000.

McMahon C, Barett B, Kowalenk N, et al: Psychological factors associated with persistent postnatal depression: past and recent relationship defence styles and the mediating role of insecure attachment style, *Journal of Affective Disorders* 84:15–24, 2005.

Miller L: Postpartum depression, *Journal of the American Medical Association* 287(6):762–765, 2002.

Murray L, Cooper PT, Wilson A, et al: Controlled trial of the short- and long-term effect of psychological treatment of postpartum depression. 2 Impact on the mother-child relationship and child outcome, *British Journal of Psychiatry* 182:420–427, 2003.

National Institute for Health and Clinical Excellence (NICE): *Antenatal and postnatal mental health: the NICE guideline on clinical management and service guidance*. Online. Available http://www.nice.org.uk/guidance/index.jsp?action=download&o=30431 3 Mar 2008, London, 2007, NICE.

National Institute for Health and Clinical Excellence (NICE): *Postnatal care. Routine postnatal care of women and their babies*, London, 2006, National Collaborating Centre For Primary Care And Royal College Of General Practitioners.

Nursing and Midwifery Council (NMC): *Midwives rules and standards*, London, 2004, NMC.

O'Connor TG, Heron J, Glover V: Antenatal anxiety predicts child behavioural/emotional problems independently of postnatal depression, *Journal of the American Academy of Child and Adolescent Psychiatry* 41(12):1470–1477, 2002.

O'Hara MW, Swain AM: Rates and risks of postpartum depression: a meta-analysis, *International Review of Psychiatry* 8:37–54, 1996.

Onozawa K, Glover V, Adams D, et al: Infant massage improves mother-infant interaction for mothers with postnatal depression, *Journal of Affective Disorders* 63:201–207, 2001.

Price A: Altered body image in pregnancy and beyond, *Britishv Journal of Midwifery* 1(3):142–146, 1993.

Price S: Midwifery care and mental health, *The Practising Midwife* 7(7): 12–14, 2004.

Price S, Lake M, Breen G, et al: The spiritual experience of high-risk pregnancy, *Journal of Obstetric, Gynecologic and Neonatal Nursing* 36:63–70, 2007.

Royal College of Midwives: *Postnatal depression soars, say midwives. Royal college of midwives, press release, 30 Apr.* Online. Available https://www.midirs. org/midirs/midweb1.nsf/Z45/m/9382E A43C4DE0E3B802572CD0038E92C October 20, 2008, 2007, Royal College of Midwives, press release, April 30.

Royal College of Psychiatrists: *Spirituality and mental health*, 2006. Online. Available http://www.rcpsych. ac.uk/mentalhealthinfo/treatments/ spiritualityandmentalhealth.aspx October 31, 2008.

Rubin R: *Maternal identity and the maternal experience*, New York, 1984, Springer Publications.

Sherr L: *The psychology of pregnancy and childbirth*, Oxford, 1995, Blackwell Science.

Snellen M: Sex and intimacy after childbirth, *Obstetrics and Gynecology* 8(3):13–15, 2006.

Stowe ZN, Hostetter AL, Newport DJ: The onset of postpartum depression: implications for clinical screening in obstetrical and primary care, *American Journal of Obstetrics and Gynecology* 192:522–526, 2005.

Swinton J: *Spirituality in mental health care: rediscovering a forgotten dimension*, London, 2001, Jessica Kingsley Publishers.

Ussher J: Depression in the postnatal period: a normal response to motherhood. In Stewart M, editor: *Pregnancy, birth and maternity care: feminist perspectives*, Edinburgh, 2004, Books for Midwives.

Way S: Episiotomy and body image, *Modern Midwife* 6(9):18–19, 1996.

Weeks NP: Serious mental illness and the midwife. In Price S, editor: *Mental health in pregnancy and childbirth*, Edinburgh, 2007, Churchill Livingstone.

World Health Organization: *WHO Guide to mental and neurological health in primary care*, London, 2004, UK Royal Society of Medicine Press.

World Health Organization: *WHO urges more investments, services for mental health*, 2008a. Online. Available http:// www.who.int/mental_health/en/ March 20, 2008.

World Health Organization: *Improving maternal mental health*, 2008b. Online. Available http://www.who.int/mental_ health/prevention/suicide/Perinatal_ depression_mmh_final.pdf October 21, 2008.

Chapter 9

Fertility control advice after birth

Trigger scenario

Mary had her third baby two days ago and she is just preparing to go home. She tells Esther, her midwife, that she does not want to become pregnant again so quickly.

Introduction

Issues relating to the control of fertility are widely related to women's health needs on a global scale. Midwives are in a strong position to promote and educate women and their partners. It has been shown that increased education of women about contraception in the postnatal period will lead to increased use (Gebreselassie et al 2008). Contraceptive use is higher in more developed countries (DESA 2003), where 69% of women aged 15–49 in relationships take precautions. According to the World Health Organization, about 80 million women every year have unintended or unwanted pregnancies (Department for International Development (DFID) 2004), and some of these are due to contraceptive failure.

The activities of a midwife include providing 'sound family planning information and advice' (NMC 2004). This means that students should have an opportunity to learn about contraception and how to give advice to women and their partners during their programmes. In order to understand the principles of fertility control, midwives should have knowledge of the menstrual

Activity

Review the menstrual cycle and physiology of the postnatal period.

Describe what specifically happens to the levels of oestrogen and progesterone after a baby is born.

Find out if there is any difference if the woman is breastfeeding her baby.

cycle and a thorough understanding of the physiology applied to the postnatal period.

When should advice be given?

The provision of fertility control advice has often been limited to a few moments prior to transfer from hospital to community or from community midwife to health visitor, or left until the postnatal examination by the general practitioner (GP) at six weeks. There is little evidence available to identify which timing is best (Hiller et al 2002). Presenting advice during the antenatal period does not appear to have a long-term effect (Smith et al 2002), though it has been recommended that discussion is started in the antenatal period to prevent causing offence in relation to religious or cultural beliefs (Schott & Henley 1996), or to ensure that the information given is retained and discussed effectively (Glasier et al 1996). However, it appears that the majority of advice is given by midwives on postnatal wards (Glasier et al 1996), with the suggestion that, as many births are unplanned, midwives should use every opportunity for health promotion purposes (Towse 2004). Current research indicates that the average time for the return of menstruation is 69 days (9 weeks), but a significant number of women will have started to menstruate before this time (Moran et al 1994).

Ovulation can return around 25 days following birth (Queenan 2004), which suggests that the current practice of giving advice early may be beneficial in preventing some unwanted pregnancies. The National Collaborating Centre for Primary Care (2006) state that fertility control advice should be given within the first seven days following birth. However, principles of woman-centred care suggest that women should be asked if they wish to discuss the provision of contraception, and their wishes should be respected if they decline at any time.

Clearly, privacy is required when giving such advice, and it should be remembered that this is not provided by curtains around beds in wards! The discussion should not be rushed as the woman should have the opportunity to assimilate and understand the information that is being given. She should also be offered the chance to ask questions and discuss any anxieties she may have. The use of information leaflets to support the advice given will assist the woman in making the decision that is right for her and her circumstances.

Activity

Find out what leaflets are available to women in your area.

Find out when these are given out, and with what verbal information.

Psychosexual issues

Recognition should be given to sensitivity surrounding the discussion of contraception after childbirth. There is evidence to suggest that the resumption of sexual behaviour following the birth of the baby may be influenced by a number of factors. For example, pain of any kind may have a negative effect on the woman's sexual desires; and the experience of birth may have resulted in tears, stitches or grazes in the vagina or perineum that will be painful (Bancroft 1995:348, Demyttenaere et al 1995). Caesarean section wounds will also be uncomfortable for a while, and the woman may not want to consider full penetrative intercourse for some time. Women may also dislike having their breasts touched due to their soreness and sensitivity (Hall 1997). In addition, some men may be put off by the production of milk for the baby, which may leak during foreplay (Bear & Tigges 1993).

Increased fatigue in the postnatal period and getting used to having a new baby in a bedroom may have an effect on parents' desires for sex. Further, there is evidence to suggest that some men have been traumatized by watching their partner in labour, and this can give them concerns about making their partner pregnant again (O'Driscoll 1994, Kitzinger 2001). Depressive illness in the woman or partner will also have a negative effect on the sexual relationship.

Some of these issues may be raised during postnatal discussion, and the midwife should be prepared to answer any questions the woman or couple may have regarding sex following birth. Advice may be given about finding alternatives to penetrative intercourse or positions where the woman may feel more comfortable. Discussion regarding timing of sex after birth will be helpful to reassure women that it is safe to resume sex when they are ready. At no time should they feel pressured into resuming sex within a certain period of time.

It is important that issues regarding sex and contraception should be raised with all women, regardless of whether they are in a stable relationship or not or whether the infant had been planned or not. Fertility control methods should be discussed with all groups of women, including teenagers (Department of Health 2003, NICE 2008). (For further information on discussing contraceptive methods with teenagers, also see Department of Health 2004.)

Choosing the correct method

In order for a woman to make the right choice regarding contraception after birth, she needs to have an understanding of all the methods available. Box 9.1 indicates the ideal characteristics of a method of contraception.

Currently available methods do not fit all these characteristics. There is evidence to suggest that a woman will often change her method of contraception after childbirth (Cwiak et al 2004). It is likely that a midwife or student may be asked about the different methods, and should give advice accordingly. The different methods fall into the categories of barrier methods, non-barrier methods and physiologic. For a comparison between the different methods and their use following birth, see Table 9.1.

Box 9.1 The ideal method of contraception (Towse 2004)

100% safe and free from side-effects
100% effective
100% reversible
Easy to use
Independent of sexual intercourse
Used by, or obviously visible, to the woman
Independent of the medical profession
Able to give protection against sexually transmitted diseases
Acceptable to both partners, all cultures and religions
Cheap and easy to distribute

Activity

Find out the differences between the combined (COC) and progestogen-only (POP) pills.

Make sure you know why the COC should not be used when breastfeeding.

Revise the different instructions women should be given for using the COC and POP effectively.

Physiologic methods

Some women may have chosen physiologic methods as contraception prior to birth, or may be interested in following these methods after birth. Physiologic methods are based on knowledge of fertility and reproduction and on self-awareness of the rhythms within a woman's cycle that indicate the time of ovulation (Cross-Sudworth 1995). For extensive descriptions of the methods that may be used, see the website of Fertility UK (www.fertilityuk.org).

The use of these methods may be more challenging in the postnatal period when the woman's hormonal levels and body functioning are adjusting. It is also a time-consuming method, and requires commitment from both partners to enhance effectiveness. The adjustment to being a new family may mean that use of these methods may be too stressful to continue. The identification of the initial time of ovulation may be difficult to assess, and women will need to be advised to take extra care at this time.

Lactational amenorrhoea

Within the physiologic method falls the lactational amenorrhoea method (LAM), or the use of breastfeeding as a method of birth spacing. When carried out successfully it is thought to be 98% effective (Labbok et al 1994, Van Look 1996, WHO 2007). The theory behind this method is that the suckling by the

Table 9.1 Methods of postpartum contraception

	Available from	Timing	Instructions	If breastfeeding	Other issues
Barrier methods					
Cap and diaphragm	GP, FPC	Fit six weeks postpartum	Instruct on use and spermicide	Yes	May need further assessment after another few weeks as body changes
Condoms and femidoms	Midwife, GP, chemists	Any time from birth	Explain use if required	Yes	Give information about emergency contraception in case of breakage
Non-barrier methods					
Combined pill (COC)	Prescription from GP, FPC	Start 21 days after birth	Additional contraception for first seven days	No	Too early may increase risk of thromboembolism. Too late may fail to inhibit first ovulation. No additional protection needed for hormonal methods if started on day 21
Progestogen-only pill (POP)	Prescription from GP, FPC	Start 21 days after birth	Additional contraception for first seven days	Yes	May start earlier but increased risk of irregular bleeding

Injectable progestogen (Depo Provera)	GP, FPC	Six weeks after birth	Additional contraception for first seven days	Yes	Earlier than six weeks more risk of irregular bleeding. Can be given if woman understands/accepts risk. Lasts 12 or 8 weeks
Implant (Implanon)	GP, FPC	Insert 21 days after birth	Additional contraception for first seven days	Yes	Lasts three years
Vaginal ring	GP, FPC	Insert 21 days after birth	Additional contraception for first seven days	Yes	
Intrauterine device and system	GP, FPC	Fit six weeks after birth unless there is a chance that woman is pregnant	May be fitted at four weeks if uterus well involuted	Yes (see right)	Conflicting evidence of risk of perforation during lactation. Lasts 3–10 years
Contraceptive patch	Prescription from GP, FPC	Start 28 days after birth	Additional contraception for first seven days	No	
Female sterilization	Referral from GP	Could be at caesarean section, if counselled, or few months after birth		Yes	Risk of failure may be higher if performed in the puerperium

infant stimulates the hypothalamus to release prolactin and oxytocin.

Activity

Describe what effect prolactin and oxytocin have on:
1. Ovulation
2. The uterus
3. Lutenizing hormone.

The success of this method is dependent on certain rules:

- Fully or nearly fully breastfeeding with intervals no longer than 4 hours during the day and 6 hours at night (Queenan 2004)
- Giving the infant no other food or drink, so no breastfeeds are missed
- The woman is not having periods after eight weeks postpartum
- It is less than six months postpartum (Labbok et al 1994, WHO Consensus Statement 1998, WHO 2007).

The basis of the six months cut-off is in relation to the number of infants who have started other foods at this time (Moloney 1998). One multicentre trial suggests that this method of contraception is 98% effective up until six months postpartum, but that this falls to 92% up to a year postpartum (Labbok et al 1997). With appropriate guidelines, women can be assured that fully breastfeeding their infant for at least six months is just as effective as other methods of contraception. The algorithm in Figure 9.1 provides the appropriate questions to ask to facilitate this method.

Making choices

Many factors influence the way women make choices about contraception. These range from their family influences to the social influences of the time, the pressures of peer groups and the age the woman was when she first had intercourse (Hepburn 1995, Matteson & Hawkins 1997). She will be influenced by the usability, availability and effectiveness of the method, as well as the point she is at in her life and whether she already has children or not. This demonstrates that the choice of contraceptive method is not necessarily a simple one.

Particular groups of women may have difficulties in relation to the limited choices available to them. For example, women who have a disability will need careful assessment with regard to which method is most suitable for them, as will women with medical conditions such as heart disease (Everett 1997). Referral to a medical practitioner or specialist nurse will need to be made to ensure counselling is carried out and the correct method is prescribed. Younger women may also benefit from the support and advice of a teenage specialist clinic. It is advisable to know the resources that are available locally to provide services to women with particular needs.

Ask the mother, or advise her to ask herself, these questions:

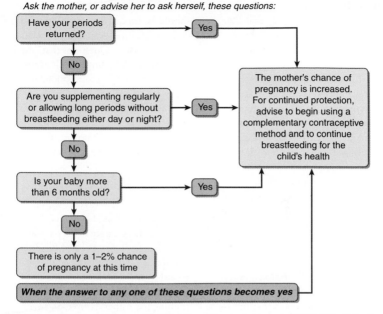

Fig. 9.1 Lactational amenorrhea method algorithm. (Source: Labbok et al 1994. © Institute of Reproductive Health, Georgetown University, Washington DC, with permission.)

Activity

Find out which fertility control services are available in your area.

Take the opportunity to visit if you can and establish links with them.

Reflection on trigger

Look back on the trigger scenario.

Mary had her third baby two days ago and she is just preparing to go home. She tells Esther, her midwife, that she does not want to become pregnant again so quickly.

The scenario describes an event that could occur daily in the postnatal period. Now that you are familiar with the issues around fertility control advice in the postnatal period you should have insight into how the scenario relates to current midwifery practice. The jigsaw model will now be used to explore the trigger scenario in more depth.

Effective communication

When considering discussion about personal information the midwife needs to think first about where the discussion is to take place to ensure privacy for the woman. In this situation the midwife also needs to assess the way that Mary has made her statement as this may indicate what she is really feeling. Questions that could be asked are: In what situation would this conversation have taken place? Is this a private environment or could the conversation be overheard? How did Mary make this statement? Were there any indicators to her feelings through her body language? What questions may Esther ask her about previous contraception? Are there questions that need to be asked in relation to Mary's relationship with her partner? What advice may Esther give at this stage? Is there written information available?

Woman-centred care

Ensuring women are placed at the centre of care involves ensuring they are included in the care, and being given appropriate information to ensure they can make the right choices. In this situation Mary should be given enough information about contraception after having a baby to ensure she will make the right choices. Questions that could be asked are: Is Mary breastfeeding her baby? What methods has she used before? Does Esther have all the appropriate information available? Are there issues in Mary's relationships or beliefs that may be affecting her choices?

Using best evidence

When giving advice midwives should use the best evidence available. In relation to contraceptive advice

this relates to when certain types should be used, their side-effects and contraindications, especially in relation to breastfeeding. Questions that could be asked are: What research is available around choice of contraception? Is Mary breastfeeding? What methods has she used before? Have these been successful for her? Does Mary have any medical condition that may affect which contraceptives are best for her?

Professional and legal issues

Midwives should always act within professional and legal guidelines. Midwives have a duty to keep up-to-date with changes in practice (NMC 2008) and this is particularly relevant with regard to advice about contraception. Questions that could be asked are: What training has Esther received on advising on contraception? Is her knowledge up-to-date? Is she working outside her sphere of knowledge? If so, whom should she refer Mary to? What professional guidelines cover this practice? What do the midwives rules of practice say about giving this information?

Team working

In all areas of practice midwives work with other team members of the multi-disciplinary team. In relation to contraception advice midwives will need to know what are the limits of their role and whom they should refer women to if further information is required. Questions that could be asked are: What are the limits of Esther's role and responsibilities? Whom could she refer

Mary to in the short term? Where else could she refer Mary in the long term? Which professionals provide care and advice in family planning clinics? Where do most women seek advice from in relation to their contraceptive needs?

Clinical dexterity

It is unlikely a midwife will require to be able to do anything on a clinical basis in order to advise on fertility control though there is potential that a woman may ask a midwife to demonstrate the use of a condom. When midwives have undertaken additional programmes of education to enable them to work in a family planning clinic they may need to develop additional skills commensurate with their role.

Models of care

In the UK midwives work within a range of models of care. In this situation it is not known whether Esther has previously been caring for Mary and is aware of her personal situation at home. As this scenario is assumed to be in a birth unit, Mary will be going home to the care of other midwives. Questions that could be asked are: Who is the most appropriate professional to advise Mary? How will the conversation be documented? Does she need to communicate any information directly to Mary's community midwife?

Safe environment

The main issue of safety in relation to conversations of this nature is to do with the confidentiality and personal space of the woman. Midwives should not discuss personal details with women where conversations may be overheard by other women or visitors. Questions that could be asked are: How will Esther ensure confidentiality is ensured? Where would the most appropriate place be on a ward to have this type of conversation? How would Esther ensure the safety of the other women and babies on the ward while she is having this conversation?

Promotes health

Principles of promoting health and wellbeing lie in ensuring that nothing is said or done that will harm the woman or her baby, but will instead contribute to her future wellbeing. This includes considering her physical, emotional and spiritual wellbeing. Questions that could be asked are: What are Mary's concerns about her wellbeing at the present time? What are her concerns for her future wellbeing? How can the correct advice around fertility control contribute to her wellbeing now and in the future? Are there potential social barriers to her wellbeing in relation to fertility control?

Further scenarios

The following scenarios enable you to consider how specific situations influence the care the midwife provides. Use the jigsaw model to explore the issues raised in each situation.

Scenario 1

Shakur is a Somali woman who has had her first baby seven days ago. She entered the country as a refugee during her pregnancy and has been diagnosed as HIV positive. Vicky, her community midwife, has come to visit Shakur, to transfer her care to the Health Visitor. Shakur's English is limited and her partner or mother-in-law have translated the information sometimes during pregnancy and are present in the home now.

Practice point

In situations where personal and private information needs to be discussed with women with poor English language skills it is not appropriate to use family members to translate the information. However it is not always easy to have an interpreter available when needed.

Questions that could be asked are:

1. Has Vicky met Shakur and her family before and built up a relationship with them?
2. Should Vicky attempt to give information about fertility control at this time?
3. Whom could she contact to arrange an interpreter for another occasion?
4. Are there any personal or religious beliefs that may affect Shakur's decisions about fertility control?
5. Will Shakur's HIV status make a difference to the choices open to her?
6. Where will Vicky document information about Shakur?
7. Should she discuss Shakur's needs with any members of the multi-professional team?

Scenario 2

Sarah goes to visit Christie at home. She is 15 years old and has had her first baby six days ago. Christie's mother answers the door to Sarah. In the hallway she asks 'Are you going to talk about contraception? You must give her something so she doesn't have any more babies.'

Practice point

In all situations the midwife has a duty of care to the mother and baby. Though Christie's mother is probably trying to be helpful, Sarah has responsibility to Christie alone and must ensure that her wishes and choices are respected. However she must also be alert to the fact that the mother may have concerns about Christie's safety.

Further questions that could be asked are:

1. Has Sarah had a relationship with this family throughout the pregnancy?
2. Does Christie's mother have a right to be present when Sarah talks to her?
3. Does Christie have a right to refuse her mother's presence?
4. How will Sarah discuss fertility control with Christie?
5. Would Sarah give different advice to Christie as a teenager than to an older woman?
6. Does Sarah need to discuss Christie's care with anyone else?
7. Where should she document the care given during the visit?
8. Does Christie need referral to anyone else for advice?

Conclusion

Knowledge of contraceptive methods is important to ensure that women are given the correct advice and support in the postnatal period. Students should take time during their midwifery education programme to observe and listen to midwives as they explore these intimate issues with women. Opportunity to practise questioning skills with peers and qualified staff will enable students to become more comfortable addressing any of the difficulties women may raise and providing appropriate information. There are many issues to consider when providing contraceptive advice to women postnatally. Women need to be assured that the person giving this advice is knowledgeable and up-to-date with contraceptive issues, and also has a good understanding of the physiological processes occurring in the postnatal period. Ultimately, a woman needs to be given advice that is appropriate for her and that will ensure any future pregnancies are planned, and not as a result of poor contraceptive choice or use. Midwives have a clear role to play in this particular aspect of health education, so must make sure that they remain informed and updated on issues of contraceptive and sexual health.

Resources

Contraceptive choices for young people: http://www.ffprhc.org.uk/admin/uploads/YoungPeople.pdf.

Erkkola R: Recent advances in hormonal contraception, *Current Opinion in Obstetrics and Gynecology* 19:547–553, 2007.

National Collaborating Centre for Primary Care (NCCPC): Postnatal care. Routine postnatal care of women and their babies, 2006. Online. Available http://www.nice.org.uk/nicemedia/pdf/CG037fullguideline.pdf October 31, 2008.

NICE: *Contraceptive services for socially disadvantaged young people – draft scope.* Online. Available http://www.nice.org.uk/guidance/index.jsp?action=download&o=42300 November 1, 2008, London, 2008, NICE.

Sexual health and relationships for young people: http://www.direct.gov.uk/en/YoungPeople/HealthAndRelationships/ConcernedAbout/DG_068631.

WHO: Family planning: a global handbook for providers. Evidence-based guidance developed through worldwide collaboration, 2007 Online. Available http://www.unfpa.org/upload/lib_pub_file/725_filename_handbook.pdf November 1, 2008.

References

Bancroft J: Sexuality and family planning. In London N, Glasier A, Gebbie A, editors: *Handbook of family planning and reproductive health care*, ed 3, Edinburgh, 1995, Churchill Livingstone.

Bear K, Tigges BB: Management strategies for promoting successful breastfeeding, *Nurse Practitioner* 18:50–60, 1993.

Cross-Sudworth FR: Natural family planning: the issues, *British Journal of Midwifery* 3(3):148–151, 1995.

Cwiak C, Gellasch T, Zieman M: Peripartum contraceptive attitudes and practices, *Contraception* 70:383–386, 2004.

Demyttenaere K, Gheldof M, Van Assche FA: Sexuality in the postpartum period: a review, *Current Opinion in Obstetrics and Gynecology* 5:81–84, 1995.

Department of Economic and Social Affairs: United Nations (DESA): *World contraceptive use*, New York, 2003, United Nations Publications.

Department for International Development (DFID): *Maternal health: factsheet*, 2004. Online. Available. http://www.dfid.gov.uk/pubs/files/maternalhealth.pdf November 1, 2008.

Department of Health: *Part six – practical tips for sexual health promotion with young people. Effective Sexual Health Promotion*, 2003. Online. Available. http://www.dh.gov.uk/assetRoot/04/07/05/58/04070558.pdf February 12, 2009.

Department of Health: *Best practice guidance for doctors and other health professionals on the provision of advice and treatment to young people under 16 on contraception, sexual and reproductive health*, 2004. Online. Available. http://www.dh.gov.uk/assetRoot/04/08/69/14/04086914.pdf February 12, 2009

Everett S: Contraception. In Andrews G, editor: *Women's sexual health*, London, 1997, Baillière Tindall.

Gebreselassie T, Rutstein SO, Mishra V: *Contraceptive use, breastfeeding, amenorrhea and abstinence during the postpartum period: an analysis of four countries. DHS Analytical Studies 14*, 2008. Online. Available http://www.measuredhs.com/pubs/pdf/AS14/AS14.pdf November 1, 2008.

Glasier AF, Logan J, McGlew TJ: Who gives advice about postpartum contraception? *Contraception* 53:217–220, 1996.

Hall J: Breastfeeding and sexuality: societal conflicts and expectations, *British Journal of Midwifery* 7(6):350–354, 1997.

Hepburn M: Factors influencing contraceptive choice. In London N, Glasier A, Gebbie A, editors: *Handbook of family planning and reproductive health care*, ed 3, Edinburgh, 1995, Churchill Livingstone.

Hiller JE, Griffith F, Jenner F: Education for contraceptive use by women after childbirth CD001863 DOI 10.1002/14651858.CD001863, *Cochrane Database of Systematic Reviews* 3(2), 2002.

Kitzinger S: Becoming a mother, *MIDIRS Midwifery Digest* 11(4): 445–447, 2001.

Labbok M, Cooney K, Coly S: *Guidelines: breastfeeding, family planning and the Lactation Amenorrhea Method (LAM)* Online. Available: http://www. linkagesproject.org/LAMCD/download/ guidelinesE.PDF October 21, 2008, Washington, Georgetown University, 1994, Institute for Reproductive Health.

Labbok MH, Hight-Laukaran V, Peterson AE, et al: Multicenter study of the Lactational Amenorrhea Method (LAM): I. Efficacy, duration, and implications for clinical application, *Contraception* 55(6):323–385, 1997.

Matteson PS, Hawkins JW: Women's patterns of contraceptive use, *Health Care for Women International* 18(5):455–466, 1997.

Moloney S: Breastfeeding as fertility suppressant: how reliable is it? *MIDIRS Midwifery Digest* 8(3):351–354, 1998.

Moran C, Alcazar L, Carvanza-Lira S, et al: Recovery of ovarian function after childbirth, lactation and sexual activity with relation to age of women, *Contraception* 50:401–407, 1994.

National Collaborating Centre for Primary Care (NCCPC): *Postnatal care. Routine postnatal care of women and their babies*, 2006. Online. Available. http://www.nice.org.uk/nicemedia/pdf/ CG037fullguideline.pdf October 31, 2008.

National Institute for Health and Clinical Excellence (NICE): *Contraceptive services for socially disadvantaged young people – draft scope* Online. Available. http://www.nice.org. uk/guidance/index.jsp?action=down load&o=42300 November 1, 2008, London, 2008, NICE.

Nursing and Midwifery Council (NMC): *Midwives rules and standards*, London, 2004, NMC.

Nursing and Midwifery Council (NMC): *The Code. Standards of conduct, performance and ethics for nurses and midwives*, London, 2008, NMC.

O'Driscoll M: Midwives, childbirth and sexuality 2: men and sex, *British Journal of Midwifery* 2(29):74, 1994.

Queenan J: Contraception and breastfeeding, *Clinical Obstetrics and Gynecology* 47(3):734–739, 2004.

Schott J, Henley A: Family planning considerations in a multiracial society, *British Journal of Midwifery* 4(8): 400–403, 1996.

Smith KB, van der Spuy ZM, Cheng L, et al: Is postpartum contraceptive advice given antenatally of value?, *Contraception* 65(3):237–243, 2002.

Towse R: Fertility and its control. In Henderson C, MacDonald S, editors: *Mayes Midwifery: a textbook for midwives*, ed 13, Edinburgh, 2004, Baillière Tindall.

Van Look P: Lactational amenorrhoea method for family planning, *Journal of Nurse Midwifery* 41(5):405–406, 1996.

WHO Consensus Statement: Lactational amenorrhoea method for family planning, *Journal of Family Planning* 17:56–59, 1998.

WHO: Family planning: a global handbook for providers: evidence-based guidance developed through worldwide collaboration, 2007. Online. Available. http://www.unfpa.org/upload/lib_pub_file/725_filename_handbook.pdf November 1, 2008.

Chapter 10

Supporting the mother to feed her baby

Trigger scenario

Emma has just given birth to her first baby. She is holding the baby with his skin naked next to hers, while Carrie, the midwife, is examining the placenta and membranes. 'I would like to feed him myself,' Emma says, 'but I don't know how to do it.'

Helping women to feed their babies

When a baby is born he is no longer fed via the placenta, the organ that maintained his needs throughout pregnancy. His nutritive requirements now need to be met by his mother, and in the developed world, this is a source of anxiety and concern for many women. They worry about whether the baby is 'getting enough' (McInnes & Chambers 2008) as well as whether they are 'doing it right' as a mother. The two main methods of feeding are with breast milk and formula. Breast milk is acknowledged as being the most appropriate source of nutrition for babies in the majority of circumstances. The World Health Organization (WHO) states that:

Breastmilk is the natural first food for babies, it provides all the energy and nutrients that the infant needs for the first months of life, and it continues to provide up to half or more of a child's nutritional needs during the second half of the first year, and up to one-third during the second year of life.

(WHO 2008)

It is recommended that women should feed their babies exclusively on breast milk for the first six months and continue breastfeeding until the child is 2 years or more (WHO/UNICEF 2003). Yet there is evidence that women in the developed world do not tend to feed their babies long term and often lack support to help them (Renfrew & Hall 2008).

Some women are influenced to breastfeed their baby, before they become pregnant, through exposure to other breastfeeding women (Hoddinott & Pill 1999). There are also societal, cultural and sexual factors involved in their choice (Hall 1997). A midwife's role is to support women in making the best choice for her and her baby, usually beginning in the antenatal period, and then to support and enable her in her chosen method. This chapter will consider the methods available to women and the midwife's role in helping women.

differentiation (Pang & Hartmann 2007). Levels of the hormone prolactin rise over pregnancy and continue to do so into the postnatal period. Levels of prolactin tend to be higher at night (Cregan et al 2002), thus breastfeeding at night should be encouraged in the postnatal period as this helps with the establishment of lactation. During pregnancy, the high levels of circulating oestrogens and progesterone prevent the breast from ejecting milk, though some colostrum may be produced in the second and third trimesters (Kent 2007).

Activity

Think about your views, knowledge and experiences of feeding babies. Do these affect your attitudes to others' choice of feeding method?

Activity

Find out where prolactin is produced and list its functions.

What may inhibit production of prolactin?

Make sure you know what colostrum is and what its constituents are.

Anatomy and physiology of breastfeeding

New advances in ultrasound technology have enabled greater understanding of the anatomy of the human breast (Ramsay et al 2004). A clear picture of the anatomy can be found at: http://www.biochem.biomedchem.uwa.edu.au/Our_People/home_pages/academic_staff/hartmann/peter_hartmann/download.

During the later stages of pregnancy a woman's body begins to prepare to produce milk for feeding (Kent 2007) which is known as secretory

After the birth of the baby and placenta, secretory activation is triggered and greater amounts of milk are secreted, accompanied by changes in the composition of the milk (Pang & Hartmann 2007). The timing for this is from 24–96 hours after birth and will vary from women to woman and birth to birth. It is thought that little milk is stored in the breast ducts as these are for transporting the milk (Ramsay et al 2004). Though it was previously believed that breast milk regulation was through a supply and demand system stimulating the production of prolactin, there is evidence that regulation is connected to how full each individual breast is and the capacity of that breast to store milk, as well as the stimulation of the infant at the breast (Daly & Hartmann 1995). However, there is further evidence that there are many physiological processes at play for breastfeeding to be initiated including the context of the early moments and days of breastfeeding (Colson 2007).

> ### Activity
>
> Find out the role of oxytocin in breastfeeding and where it is produced.

Reflexes

The release of the milk by the mother is a neurohormonal reflex called the 'let-down reflex'. Sucking at the breast will initiate the reflex, but this may also be stimulated by the mother seeing, smelling, touching or hearing her baby (Ackerman 2004). Initially the reflex may be unconditioned but will become conditioned to the baby over time. However, the let-down reflex may also be prevented by the mother becoming anxious or stressed (Johnson & Taylor 2006).

The baby also has primitive reflexes in relation to feeding:

- The rooting reflex is stimulated by touching the cheek of the newborn baby, causing the baby to turn towards the touch and usually to open his mouth

- The sucking reflex will be stimulated by placing something into the baby's mouth (Schott and Rossor 2003).

Colson et al (2003, 2008) highlight that primitive reflexes may give clues to feeding behaviour and be stimulated or hindered by the positioning of the mother.

> ### Activity
>
> Observe the rooting and sucking reflex in a newborn baby.
> Think about how knowledge of these reflexes in mother and baby would impact on care.

Breast milk

Breast milk is considered to be the ideal form of milk for individual babies as it is easy for the baby to absorb. It has the ideal constituents for an infant's nutrition for the first six months of life and it gives immunological protection (Michaelsen 2003). It also varies:

- With the time of day
- With the stage of lactation
- In response to maternal nutrition
- According to the individual mother and baby dyad (Inch 2004).

Benefits of breastfeeding

Breastfeeding has been shown to be beneficial for both mother and baby.

In comparison to babies who are formula fed, babies who are fully breastfed for 4–6 months are less likely to get:

- Gastroenteritis
- Respiratory infections
- Otitis media
- Urinary tract infection
- Necrotizing enterocolitis
- Atopic disease (Stanley et al 2007).

Further, there are indications that babies fed on formula may be more at risk of diabetes, inflammatory bowel disease, coeliac disease, childhood leukaemia, and dental occlusion (MIDIRS 2007).

Mothers may also benefit from breastfeeding through:

- Being less likely to develop breast cancer and ovarian cancer
- Reduced risk of postnatal depression
- Reduced risk of type 2 diabetes (Stanley et al 2007).

Guidance for supporting women

Midwives can help women breastfeed by having a positive attitude, keeping hands off when helping with positioning baby at the breast, being aware of women's thoughts and feelings and spending time with them. The UNICEF *Baby Friendly Initiative* was devised to provide maternity services with guidance to ensure the ideal care is given to support women. They created ten steps that would indicate that the service is shown to be ideal (WHO/ UNICEF 1989).

The ten steps are listed in Box 10.1.

These ten steps apply to all areas where babies are cared for, which includes postnatal wards, neonatal units and in the community. Maternity units can achieve 'baby friendly' accreditation following an assessment of their implementation of the ten steps.

Activity

Is your unit 'baby friendly? If not, in what areas does the service not adhere to the above list and why?

List any problems which could arise with having 'baby friendly' status.

Define 'demand' feeding.

A Cochrane review into the types of support available to breastfeeding women, examining 34 studies which included about 30 000 women, showed that both professional and lay support and the two combined, could be effective in areas where breastfeeding rates were not high (Britton et al 2007). A qualitative synthesis of women's experiences of support (McInnes & Chambers 2008) concluded that:

- The relationship between the mother and professional were important, with positive support as being encouraging, non-judgmental, sympathetic, patient and understanding.
- Characteristics of unhelpful support were being 'directive or authoritarian',

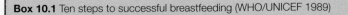

Box 10.1 Ten steps to successful breastfeeding (WHO/UNICEF 1989)

1. Have a written breastfeeding policy that is routinely communicated to all healthcare staff.
2. Train all healthcare staff in skills necessary to implement this policy.
3. Inform all pregnant women about the benefits and management of breastfeeding.
4. Help mothers initiate breastfeeding soon after birth.
5. Show mothers how to breastfeed, and how to maintain lactation even if they should be separated from their infants.
6. Give newborn infants no food or drink other than breast milk, unless medically indicated.
7. Practise rooming in – allow mothers and infants to remain together 24 hours a day.
8. Encourage breastfeeding on demand.
9. Give no artificial teats or dummies to breastfeeding infants.
10. Foster the establishment of breastfeeding support groups and refer mothers to them on discharge from the hospital.

'taking over', giving encouragement without practical advice, and conflicting advice.

- Formula supplementation, demand feeding, poor weight gain and maternal diet were more likely to lead to conflicting advice.
- Having skilled help was significant, but women disliked a 'physically intrusive, distressing and embarrassing 'hands-on' approach.' Women found difficulty in achieving positioning and latching the baby on when it had previously been 'done' by the health professional.
- Time pressures were identified as a source of difficulties with help not being 'offered pro-actively' and women feeling 'left to get on with it'.
- Women identified a perceived 'medicalisation of breastfeeding' with professionals 'anxiety bout the 'need to measure' how much milk the baby was getting.'
- The public nature of postnatal wards and neonatal units with women identifying 'breastfeeding in public as an issue'.
- Women in supportive family and social networks were more likely to overcome feeding difficulties. Peers and group support were also important for successful breastfeeding.

Skin-to-skin contact

It has been shown that placing the naked baby next to the mother's skin (skin-to-skin contact) as soon as possible after birth is beneficial for both mother and baby on a number of levels. A Cochrane review of 30 studies (Moore et al 2007), involving 1925 mothers and babies, showed that babies who had close contact after birth:

- Interacted more with their mothers
- Stayed warmer
- Cried less
- Were more likely to breastfeed
- Breastfeed longer.

Skin-to-skin care is recommended in the NICE intrapartum guidelines (National Institute for Health and Clinical Excellence (NICE) 2007:21) and should be offered to women, whether they intend to breastfeed their baby or not. Unfortunately in many units the lack of time available may prevent this from being offered for a sustained length of time. Though skin-to-skin care may be suggested as beneficial for breastfeeding, research has demonstrated that in practice women may prefer to keep babies clothed (Colson et al 2003).

How to help a woman breastfeed

The basis of helping women to feed is to facilitate them to do this with their baby, rather than 'taking over' and 'doing it to them' (McInnes & Chambers 2008).

Preparation

- As women may be feeding their baby for 30–60 minutes they should be encouraged to consider what they need to have prepared around them prior to feeding their baby.
- As feeding the baby may make the woman feel thirsty, she should have a drink nearby.
- Assess whether the baby needs his nappy to be changed before a feed to ensure he is comfortable.

Comfort

- As women may be feeding their baby for 30–60 minutes they should be encouraged to empty their bladder prior to feeding. The release of oxytocin may cause the uterus to contract and make a woman feel uncomfortable if her bladder is full.
- The woman should consider where she will be most comfortable to feed so that she can relax and enjoy the feed in comfort.

Position of mother

There has been specific guidance for how a mother and her baby should be positioned for feeding (Ackerman 2004, Inch 2004). However, it is suggested that this prescriptive approach may not be helpful for everyone (Colson 2005). Suzanne Colson states that the appropriate maternal posture is:

- One that the mother says is comfortable
- Where there is no neck strain, shoulders are relaxed and all body parts are supported
- Pain free, sustainable for a long period of time.

She goes on to state that:

1. Since all mothers' bodies are different, there is not one posture that will fit all needs.
2. Mothers easily find the right posture for their own needs and comfort when routine suggestions are avoided.
3. Comfortable, sustainable postures will change and evolve throughout the breastfeeding time span. Initially, they may change from feed to feed or daily (Colson 2005:30).

Position of baby

Feeding positions in Colson's (2005) *Biological Nurturing* approach are defined 'as those where the entire frontal aspect of the baby's body is in close juxtaposition with a maternal body contour'. She indicates that potentially there may be 200 positions in which the baby could lie (Colson 2005). In practice, when women are outside the privacy of home, some of these positions may be less practical.

The NICE postnatal guidelines (NICE 2006) advise that women should be given certain information as indicators of good attachment and positioning and success of breastfeeding (see Box 10.2).

Helping women with formula feeding

As with breastfeeding, women who choose to feed their baby with formula also need guidance and support from midwives. NICE (2006:26) states that these women:

should be taught how to make feeds using correct, measured quantities of formula, as based on the manufacturer's instructions, and how to cleanse and sterilise feeding bottles and teats and how to store formula milk.

Activity

Find out about the different formula milks that are available in the shops.
Are there any differences between them?
Make sure you understand the difference between formula milk and breast milk.

Equipment and sterilizing

There are a number of different styles and types of infant feeding bottles on the market and numerous types of teats available. In addition there are ready-made up feeds, which tend to be

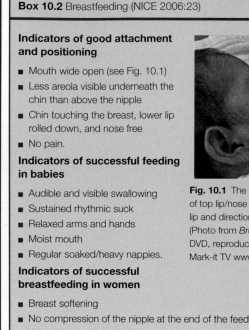

Box 10.2 Breastfeeding (NICE 2006:23)

Indicators of good attachment and positioning

- Mouth wide open (see Fig. 10.1)
- Less areola visible underneath the chin than above the nipple
- Chin touching the breast, lower lip rolled down, and nose free
- No pain.

Indicators of successful feeding in babies

- Audible and visible swallowing
- Sustained rhythmic suck
- Relaxed arms and hands
- Moist mouth
- Regular soaked/heavy nappies.

Indicators of successful breastfeeding in women

- Breast softening
- No compression of the nipple at the end of the feed
- Woman feels relaxed and sleepy.

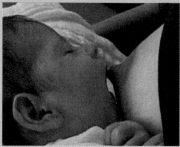

Fig. 10.1 The wide gape. Note the proximity of top lip/nose to nipple, position of bottom lip and direction that nipple enters the mouth (Photo from *Breastfeeding – The Essentials* DVD, reproduced with kind permission of Mark-it TV www.markittelevision.com).

more costly. Women will probably be influenced by cost when purchasing equipment. It is suggested that women will require:

- Six bottles with lids, covers and teats to cover a 24-hour period.
- Sterilizing equipment to ensure the bottles are sterile prior to putting the feed inside and prevent introducing infection to the baby.
- Bottle and teat brushes (non-metallic) to ensure effective cleaning of the bottles and teats. Metal brushes will

be affected by the chemicals used in sterililizing.

- Sterilizable tongs or tweezers for adding the top and teat without using hands.
- Plastic spatula or leveller in case these are not in the formula packet.
- A kettle or means to boil water as feeds need to be made up with boiled water (Johnson & Taylor 2006:358).

Concerns about potential micro-organisms that are present in formula milk have led to the Department of

Health (2007:01) to issue the message to health carers to warn parents:

that powdered infant formula is not sterile and good hygiene practices are essential in preparing and storing feeds made from powdered formula. (p.1)

It is important that women are therefore taught the principles of hygiene and sterilization of equipment for the protection of the baby.

Activity

Find out about the different types of sterilizers, sterilizing solutions and tablets available on the market.

The Department of Health (2007) instructions are as follows:

- Wash hands thoroughly before cleaning and sterilizing feeding equipment.
- Wash feeding and preparation equipment thoroughly in hot soapy water.
- Bottle and teat brushes should be used to scrub inside and outside of bottles and teats to ensure that all remaining feed is removed.
- After washing feeding equipment rinse it thoroughly under the tap.
- If using a commercial sterilizer, follow manufacturer's instructions.
- If your bottles are suitable for sterilizing by boiling: fill a large pan with water and completely submerge all feeding equipment, ensuring there are no air bubbles trapped;

cover the pan and boil for at least 10 minutes, making sure the pan does not boil dry. Keep the pan covered until equipment is needed.

- Wash hands thoroughly and clean the surface around the sterilizer before removing equipment.
- It is best to remove the bottles just before they are used.
- If the bottles are not being used immediately, they should be fully assembled with the teat and lid in place to prevent the inside of the sterilized bottle and the inside and outside of the teat from being contaminated. (pp 1–2)

Making up a feed

Feeds should be made up when they are needed and not stored, due to the risk of growth of micro-organisms. This usually involves placing a scoop (that is usually provided with the individual packets of feed) of dry formula to about 30 ml or one fluid ounce of cooled, boiled water. The powder should not be used beyond the packet expiry date. The instructions for making an infant feed are as follows (Department of Health 2007:03):

1. Clean the surface thoroughly on which to prepare the feed.
2. Wash hands with soap and water and then dry.
3. Boil fresh tap water in a kettle. Alternatively bottled water that is suitable for infants can be used for making up feeds and should be boiled in the same way as tap water.

4. **Important:** Allow the boiled water to cool to *no less than 70°C*. This means in practice using water that has been left covered, for less than 30 minutes after boiling.

5. Pour the amount of boiled water required into the sterilized bottle.

6. Add the exact amount of formula as instructed on the label, always using the scoop provided with the powdered formula by the manufacturer. Adding more or less powder than instructed could make the baby ill.

7. Re-assemble the bottle following manufacturer's instructions.

8. Shake the bottle well to mix the contents.

9. Cool quickly to feeding temperature by holding under a running tap, or placing in a container of cold water.

10. Check the temperature by shaking a few drops onto the inside of your wrist – it should feel lukewarm, not hot.

11. Discard any feed that has not been used within 2 hours.

Amount of feed

As with breastfeeding, women may practise 'demand' feeding with an infant, which involves feeding when the baby is hungry. In practice this will probably be every 3 to 4 hours. Initially a 30 ml amount may be enough; however a further 30 ml may be made up should the baby finish this amount, and the amounts increased over subsequent feeds. Documentation of how much the baby is taking and the frequency should be made initially, while feeding patterns are being established. In addition women should be aware that the baby's stool will be firmer than that of a breastfeeding baby and may smell stronger.

Activity

Find out about cup feeding. What equipment is required and when is this recommended?

Reflection on trigger scenario

Look back on the trigger scenario.

Emma has just given birth to her first baby. She is holding the baby with his skin naked next to hers, while Carrie, the midwife, is examining the placenta and membranes. 'I would like to feed him myself,' Emma says, 'but I don't know how to do it.'

The scenario describes an event that could occur in any midwifery situation. Now that you are familiar with the issues around supporting a woman to feed her baby you should have insight into how the scenario relates to current midwifery practice. The jigsaw model will now be used to explore the trigger scenario in more depth.

Effective communication

During the antenatal period Emma will have received a considerable amount of information about infant feeding, in both written and verbal forms. She may have also found out information for herself from reading, from internet information and from friends and family. How this information will have been presented will have an impact on Emma's understanding and knowledge about feeding. In this scenario, straight away following birth, how Emma has experienced birth will also have an impact on her receptivity at this time. In responding to Emma's statement, Carrie will need to consider verbal clues and body language to establish how Emma is feeling about feeding. Other questions that could be asked are: What knowledge does Emma have already? How will Carrie establish this? What information will Carrie give her? Are there any areas of stress around Carrie's workload that may prevent her from communicating appropriately? What are Carrie's views of feeding that may impact on how the information is communicated to Emma? Where will Carrie document information about how and when the baby was fed?

Woman-centred care

In order to provide woman-centred care the midwife will need to explore the woman's hopes and expectations around her chosen method of feeding. She might also explore what support the woman has and if she has any experience of her chosen method. In this situation, both the needs of Emma and the baby need to be considered. Questions that could be asked are: How may Carrie ensure Emma's specific needs are reflected in the plan of care for herself and the baby at this time? How will Carrie establish what these needs are? How can Carrie make best use of the support networks that Carrie has available to her?

Using best evidence

There is a great deal of evidence available to inform both the woman and the midwife of the most appropriate ways to initiate breastfeeding. Evidence is available in a range of formats, from professional, maternity unit and breastfeeding support group leaflets to NICE guidance and systematic reviews of the available evidence. In particular, the hour after birth is a time when the baby is often alert and ready to feed. In this scenario Emma has already been holding her baby next to her skin. Questions that could be asked are: What is the evidence around initiating breastfeeding immediately after birth? What national and international guidance is available? Is there any evidence about the benefits of feeding a baby as soon as possible after birth? What senses does the baby use to locate the nipple and attach itself to the breast?

Professional and legal issues

Midwives have professional and legal accountability both to their professional body and to their employer. They have a duty of care to the mother and her baby. Questions that could be asked are: What do the Midwives rules and standards (NMC 2004) say about the practices of infant feeding? What aspects of the Code (NMC 2008) are relevant to the midwife supporting a woman to breastfeed? What are the expectations of the unit/trust in which Emma works in relation to employees supporting infant feeding? Does it have baby friendly status and does that impact on the care given?

Team working

Midwives can work autonomously but also with other midwives and professionals to provide care for breastfeeding women. In this situation Carrie should be able to support Emma to breastfeed her baby. However, there my be others who could provide additional support with infant feeding whilst Emma is in hospital. Questions that could be asked are: Who could support Emma as she gains confidence with breastfeeding her baby? Which lay breastfeeding support groups work in the hospital? Who would be available to support Emma when she goes home? How is this information communicated to Emma? What are the processes midwives need to follow in order to access additional support for breastfeeding women?

Clinical dexterity

In this situation the dexterity lies in not doing anything, but supporting Emma to feed the baby herself. Carrie may help by assisting Emma into the most comfortable position prior to starting feeding. Carrie needs to be able to recognize when the baby has latched

well onto the breast. Questions that could be asked are: How can Emma be made comfortable? Does she need to empty her bladder prior to feeding? Are there any assessments that Carrie needs to make of Emma prior to making her comfortable to feed? Is the environment appropriate to enable Emma to feed?

Models of care

It is not clear from the scenario which model Carrie is working in. However, this situation could apply in any model of care. In a home situation Carrie may be working with another midwife who may be in a position to help tidy equipment while Carrie helps Emma feed. Questions that could be asked are: Is supporting feeding Carrie's role? Is there another member of the team who could help Emma with feeding? How does continuity of care enhance the initiation and continuation of breastfeeding? Should a woman stay in hospital to establish feeding or return home as soon as possible? How do members of the maternity care team communicate with each other about the support and advice they have provided to Emma?

Safe environment

Carrie should ensure that prior to supporting Emma to feed that the environment is safe for her to do so. Sometimes labour ward beds are high and narrow, which would make holding and feeding her baby both difficult and potentially unsafe. Questions that could be asked are: Can Emma be encouraged to move into a comfortable position that will be safe for her and her baby? Does Carrie need to consider moving Emma to a safer position? Are there any hazards in the environment? Can Carrie move safely around the environment? How does Carrie protect Emma's privacy and dignity throughout the first feed?

Promotes health

There is no question from the evidence as summarized by MIDIRS (2007) that breastfeeding is a healthy activity for both mother and baby. However, it cannot be assumed that women and their families are aware of the latest evidence in this area. Carrie may also consider other issues around the promotion of health whilst she has the opportunity to be with Emma in this focused way. Questions that could be asked are: What information should Carrie give Emma about breastfeeding? How will Emma's self-esteem be promoted? What other messages can Carrie convey to Emma at this time. What messages can Carrie convey to Emma's birth partner that might facilitate breastfeeding?

Further scenarios

The following scenarios enable you to consider how specific situations influence the care the midwife provides. Use the jigsaw model to explore the issues raised in each situation.

Scenario 1

Vanessa visits Maria at home. Maria had her baby six days ago. Up until today she has been breastfeeding her baby but has decided now to feed with artificial milk.

Practice point

Women may decide to change to artificial feeding at any time and support should be given in their choice. However it is appropriate to establish why they have decided to change their minds as it may be due to an issue that the midwife will be able to help with. It may be an opportunity to correct misconceptions about how much milk the baby is getting or why the baby is feeding frequently.

Further questions may be:

1. What questions will Vanessa ask Maria?
2. What factors could have made her stop feeding the baby?
3. Is it appropriate to observe Maria feeding the baby?
4. What advice will Vanessa give about formula feeding?
5. What equipment does Maria have and what does she need?
6. What documentation will be required?

Scenario 2

Laura has had her baby two days ago and is trying to breastfeed. However, the baby appears not to be latching on well and slipping off the breast. On examination it is noted that the baby has a significant tongue tie.

Practice point

In the NICE postnatal guideline (NICE 2006) in cases of tongue tie (ankyloglossia), it is recommended that the first course of action is to assess feeding and establish if position and attachment are appropriate. If the baby still does not feed then frenulotomy may be required.

Further questions that could be asked are:

1. Is Laura's baby attaching appropriately?
2. How will the midwife assess if attachment is correct?
3. What is frenulotomy?
4. Who carries this out in your locality?
5. What is the success rate in relation to breastfeeding?
6. What information may be given to Laura about tongue tie and frenulotomy?
7. What assessments may be made following frenulotomy?
8. Where will this be recorded?

Conclusion

Most babies initiate feeding soon after birth. What and how they will be fed will be the mother's choice which will be influenced by a range of cultural, social, and practical issues. However, for most babies, breastfeeding is the most appropriate form of nutrition, providing all of his nutritive requirements until 6 months of age. A midwife's role is to enable a woman to make the right choice of feeding method for her and her baby, and to enable her and support her in that choice. This involves giving appropriate, factual information as well as practical guidance on how to feed the baby.

Resources

Baby Friendly Initiative. http://www.babyfriendly.org.uk/page.asp?page=11.

Biological Nurturing. http://www.biologicalnurturing.com/index.html.

La Leche League International: http://www.llli.org/.

NHS breastfeeding website: http://www.breastfeeding.nhs.uk/en/fe/page.asp?n1=5.

'Recipe for nurturing' leaflet. http://www.biologicalnurturing.com/images/pdf/Poster%20for%20web%20site-locked.pdf.

World Health Organization website: http://www.who.int/topics/breastfeeding/en/.

References

Ackerman B: Infant feeding. In Henderson C, MacDonald S, editors: *Mayes midwifery: a textbook for midwives*, ed 13, Oxford, 2004, Baillière Tindall.

Britton C, McCormick FM, Renfrew MJ, et al: Support for breastfeeding mothers CD001141, *Cochrane Database of Systematic Reviews*(1), 2007.

Colson S: Maternal breastfeeding positions: have we go it right? (2), *The Practising Midwife* 8(11):29–32, 2005.

Colson S: The physiology of lactation revisited, *The Practising Midwife* 10(10):14–19, 2007.

Colson S, de Rooy L, Hawdon JM: Biological nurturing increases duration of breastfeeding for a vulnerable cohort, *MIDIRS Midwifery Digest* 13(1):92–97, 2003.

Colson S, Meek JH, Hawdon JM: Optimal positions for the release of primitive neonatal reflexes stimulating breastfeeding, *Early Human Development* 84(7):441–449, 2008.

Cregan MD, Mitoulas LR, Hartmann PE: Milk prolactin, feed volume and duration between feeds in women breastfeeding their full-term infants over a 24 h period, *Experimental Physiology* 87(2):207–214, 2002.

Daly SE, Hartmann P: Infant demand and milk supply. Part 1: infant demand and milk production in lactating women, *Journal of Human Lactation* 11(1):21–26, 1995.

Department of Health: *Guidance for health professionals on safe preparation, storage and handling of powdered infant formula*, 2007. Online. Available http://www.dh.gov.uk/en/Healthcare/ Maternity/Maternalandinfantnutrition/ DH_4123674 October 31, 2008.

Hall J: Breastfeeding and sexuality: societal conflicts and expectations, *British Journal of Midwifery* 5(6): 350–354, 1997.

Hoddinott P, Pill R: Qualitative study of decisions about infant feeding among women in east end of London, *British Medical Journal* 318:30–34, 1999.

Inch S: Feeding. In Fraser DM, Cooper MA, editors: *Myles textbook for midwives*, ed 14, Edinburgh, 2004, Churchill Livingstone.

Johnson R, Taylor W: *Skills for midwifery practice*, ed 2, Edinburgh, 2006, Elsevier.

Kent JC: How breastfeeding works, *Journal of Midwifery and Women's Health* 52(6):564–570, 2007.

McInnes RJ, Chambers JA: Supporting breastfeeding mothers: qualitative synthesis, *Journal of Advanced Nursing* 62(4):407–427, 2008.

MIDIRS: *Informed choice initiative. neonatal and infant care 7: breastfeeding or bottle feeding for professionals*, Bristol, 2007, MIDIRS.

Moore ER, Anderson GC, Bergman N: Early skin-to-skin contact for mothers and their healthy newborn infants,

Cochrane Database of Systematic Reviews Issue 3(CD003519), 2007. DOI: 10.1002/14651858.CD003519. pub2.

National Institute for Health and Clinical Excellence (NICE): *Postnatal care. Routine postnatal care of women and their babies*, 2006. Online. Available http://www.nice.org.uk/nicemedia/pdf/CG037fullguideline.pdf October 31, 2008.

National Institute for Health and Clinical Excellence (NICE): *Intrapartum care of healthy women and their babies during childbirth*, London, 2007, RCOG Press.

Nursing and Midwifery Council (NMC): *Midwives rules and standards*, London, 2004, NMC.

Nursing and Midwifery Council (NMC): *The Code. Standards of conduct, performance and ethics for nurses and midwives*, London, 2008, NMC.

Pang WW, Hartmann PE: Initiation of human lactation: secretory differentiation and secretory activation, *Journal of Mammary Gland Biology and Neoplasia* 12(4):1703–1709, 2007.

Ramsay DT, Kent JC, Owens RA, et al: Ultrasound imaging of milk ejection in the breast of lactating women, *Pediatrics* 113(2):361–367, 2004.

Renfrew M, Hall D: Enabling women to breast feed, *British Medical Journal* 337:a1570, 2008.

Schott JM, Rossor MN: The grasp and other primitive reflexes, *Journal of Neurology, Neurosurgery & Psychiatry* 74:558–560, 2003.

Stanley I, Chung M, Raman G: *Breastfeeding and maternal and infant health outcomes in developed countries*, Evidence Report/Technology Assessment, Number 153., Boston, MA, 2007, Agency for Healthcare Research and Quality.

WHO/UNICEF: *Protecting, promoting and supporting breast-feeding: the special role of maternity services. A Joint WHO/UNICEF Statement*, Geneva, 1989, WHO.

WHO/UNICEF: *Global strategy for infant and young child feeding*, Geneva, 2003, WHO.

WHO: Exclusive breastfeeding. Online. Available http://www.who.int/nutrition/topics/exclusive_breastfeeding/en/ October 27, 2008.

Index